Facilitated Stretching

Second Edition

Robert E. McAtee
and Jeff Charland

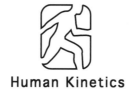

Human Kinetics

Library of Congress Cataloging-in-Publication Data

McAtee, Robert E., 1948-
    Facilitated stretching / by Robert E. McAtee. -- 2nd ed.
        p.   cm.
    Includes bibliographical references (p.   ) and index.
        ISBN 0-7360-0066-6
        1. Stretching exercises--Popular works.   2. Athletes.   3. Physical
    therapy--Popular works.   I. Title.
    RA781.63.M33   1999
    613.7'11--DC21   98-37474
                                                                       CIP

ISBN-10: 0-7360-0066-6
ISBN-13: 978-0-7360-0066-6

Acquisitions Editor: Loarn Robertson; **Developmental Editors:** Holly Gilly, Laura Casey Mast; **Assistant Editor:** Leigh LaHood; **Copyeditor:** Allen Gooch; **Proofreader:** Erin Cler; **Indexer:** Marie Rizzo; **Graphic Designer:** Nancy Rasmus; **Graphic Artist:** Kathleen Boudreau-Fuoss; **Photo Editor:** Tom Roberts; **Cover Designer:** Keith Blomberg; **Photographer (cover):** Tom Roberts; **Photographer (interior):** Figures 3.3, 3.4, 5.8, and 5.19 by Wendy Pearce Nelson; all other photos by Tom Roberts; **Illustrators:** Beth Young, Keith Blomberg; **Models:** Scott Adair, Randy Beech, Tay Cambell, Matt Carpenter, Jeff Charland, Terry Devlin, Roger Francisco, Brian Hawn, Elizabeth Holder, Philip Natividad, Shanese Simpson, and Jill Trenary; **Printer:** United Graphics

Human Kinetics books are available at special discounts for bulk purchase. Special editions or book excerpts can also be created to specification. For details, contact the Special Sales Manager at Human Kinetics.

Printed in the United States of America   10

Human Kinetics
Web site: www.HumanKinetics.com

United States: Human Kinetics, P.O. Box 5076, Champaign, IL 61825-5076
800-747-4457
e-mail: humank@hkusa.com

Canada: Human Kinetics, 475 Devonshire Road Unit 100, Windsor, ON N8Y 2L5
800-465-7301 (in Canada only)
e-mail: orders@hkcanada.com

Europe: Human Kinetics, 107 Bradford Road, Stanningley, Leeds LS28 6AT, United Kingdom
+44 (0) 113 255 5665
e-mail: hk@hkeurope.com

Australia: Human Kinetics, 57A Price Avenue, Lower Mitcham, South Australia 5062
08 8277 1555
e-mail: liaw@hkaustralia.com

New Zealand: Human Kinetics, Division of Sports Distributors NZ Ltd., P.O. Box 300 226 Albany
North Shore City, Auckland
0064 9 448 1207
e-mail: info@humankinetics.co.nz

To my mentors, colleagues, and students,
without whom this book would not have been possible.

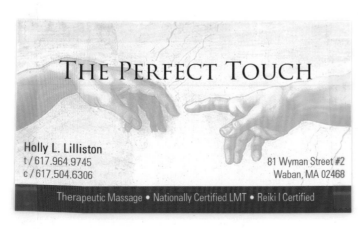

Contents

Preface

Flexibility and coordination make it easier to accomplish any task that requires the use of muscles. They are major components of optimum athletic performance and also play an important role in our daily lives outside of athletics. Flexibility and coordination are critical to preventing injuries, whether on the playing field, in the warehouse, or in front of the computer. Overuse injuries, also known as repetitive stress injuries, occur in part because of lack of flexibility caused by tight muscles.

Facilitated stretching is an easy way to maintain or improve flexibility and coordination. It can be done with a partner or by yourself and can easily be incorporated into an existing stretching program.

This second edition of *Facilitated Stretching* has been changed significantly from the first to reflect my improved understanding of the technique and its applications beyond athletics. This edition has been reorganized to make it easier to use, to broaden the scope of stretches presented, and to update you on the latest research available on PNF (proprioceptive neuromuscular facilitation) stretching techniques. You'll find 154 new photographs and illustrations, and stretches for additional muscle groups, including the cervical region. Many of the stretches from the first edition have been modified to make them more effective and easier to do.

I believe the most significant change in this second edition is the emphasis on self-stretching. For any flexibility program to be effective, it must be practiced regularly, not just during occasional visits to a sports therapist or trainer. For this reason, I've expanded the number of self-stretches and modified many of those from the first edition. Many of these modifications have been inspired by students and colleagues.

You'll also find a greater emphasis throughout the book on the active role the stretcher must take for facilitated stretching techniques to help him or her achieve optimum flexibility and coordination. To this end, I've expanded the discussion of biomechanics and stabilization for both the stretcher and the partner.

Jeff Charland has expanded his chapter on the use of PNF techniques in a physical therapy setting. We hope this will give you a broader understanding of the scope of PNF in a rehabilitative program. Jeff has also contributed to the section on biomechanics and has worked with me on fine-tuning many of the new stretches.

In a separate appendix, I've added new material for therapists that discusses facilitated stretching in conjunction with manual soft tissue therapy to restore range of motion lost because of accident or injury. The blend of stretching and hands-on work is amazingly effective in reducing scar tissue and adhesions to improve pain-free motion.

I've also placed the research on PNF stretching techniques in an appendix for those readers who would like a more scientific and in-depth look at how and why PNF techniques work.

In the years since the first edition was released, I've had the honor of teaching thousands of people how to incorporate facilitated stretching into their lives. I've learned a lot from them in the process. The distillation of that learning is in these pages. This second edition is more complete, easier to use, and a truer reflection of the benefits available from PNF techniques.

If you're a sports therapist, athletic trainer, sports physician, coach, or competitive athlete, you'll find valuable information here for optimizing performance. If you lead an active life, or are just beginning a fitness program, you'll find that these techniques will help you gain increased flexibility and coordination, which can help prevent injuries and improve your enjoyment of your chosen activities.

Acknowledgments

No book can be written and produced without the help of many people.

Several people read the manuscript and offered suggestions that greatly improved its organization, clarity, and usefulness. For their careful reading and thoughtful comments, I thank Keith Grant, Ed Reedholm, Julie Leshay, Charna Rosenholtz, Paul Witt, and Mike Stephens.

Thanks to Loarn Robertson, PhD, my acquisitions editor at Human Kinetics. He guided me through the early stages of the manuscript, helping to shape and focus it. My appreciation also goes to Laura Casey Mast and Holly Gilly, my developmental editors, and to Leigh LaHood, assistant editor. They took into account my teaching and travel schedule in setting manuscript deadlines, scheduling photo shoots, and handling the myriad details that went into the production of this book. I'd also like to thank the rest of the Human Kinetics family who had a hand in the development, production, and marketing of the book.

Bob McAtee, LMT, CSCS
Colorado Springs, Colorado

PART 1

Understanding PNF Stretching

Most of us know that stretching is an important part of training for any sport. Beyond sport, stretching is useful for maintaining general flexibility for daily activities and as preventive maintenance in repetitive motion activities.

There are many ways to stretch, from the overall stretches we do naturally to specific techniques found in the many books available today. Over the past 15 years, PNF (proprioceptive neuromuscular facilitation) stretching has gained popularity, especially in the athletic community and increasingly with the general public. PNF stretching is but one aspect of PNF, which is a complex and highly effective physical therapy technique. PNF stretching uses an isometric contraction prior to the stretch to achieve greater gains than from stretching alone. PNF stretching is generally done passively; that is, the physical therapist does the stretching for the patient.

Facilitated stretching is based on PNF principles and techniques but is an *active* form of stretching, in which the stretcher does most or all of the work. When a partner is involved, the partner's job is to monitor and direct the stretcher's activity.

Facilitated stretching can bring about dramatic gains in flexibility in a very short time because of the creative use of several built-in neurological mechanisms to optimize a muscle's ability to lengthen. In chapter 1, you'll find a brief account of how PNF developed and learn the neurophysiological basics of PNF theory on which facilitated stretching is based. In chapters 2 and 3, you will learn how to do facilitated stretching. A thorough grounding in the *why* of PNF theory will make the *how* easier in daily practice.

Historical Development of PNF

Proprioceptive neuromuscular facilitation (PNF) is a treatment technique developed in the late 1940s and early 1950s by Herman Kabat, MD, PhD, and two physical therapists, Margaret "Maggie" Knott and Dorothy Voss. Kabat, a neurophysiologist, based much of the theoretical structure of PNF on the work of Sir Charles Sherrington, whose research in the early to mid-1900s helped develop a model for how the neuromuscular system operates (Sherrington 1947).

Kabat believed that the principles of neurophysiological development and Sherrington's laws of irradiation, successive induction, and reciprocal innervation should be applied in the rehabilitation of polio patients with paralysis. Before the development of PNF techniques, paralyzed patients had been rehabilitated using methods that emphasized "one motion, one joint, one muscle at a time" (Voss, Ionta, and Myers 1985). With backing from industrialist Henry Kaiser, Kabat founded the Kabat-Kaiser Institute (KKI) in Washington, DC, in 1946 and began working with paralysis patients to find combinations and patterns of movement that were consistent with neurophysiological theory. By 1951, Kabat and Knott had identified and established nine techniques for rehabilitating muscles.

Physical therapist Dorothy Voss became interested in PNF in 1950, learning from and working with Knott. She was subsequently hired as Knott's assistant in 1952. Voss and Knott realized that PNF was more than a system for the treatment of paralysis; it was a new way of thinking about and using movement and therapeutic exercise.

In 1952 Knott and Voss began presenting workshops to train other physical therapists in PNF methods. By 1954 they were conducting two-week trainings, and in 1956 they published the first edition of *Proprioceptive Neuromuscular Facilitation*.

During the 1960s, PNF courses became available through physical therapy departments at several universities, and their popularity continued to grow. PNF techniques are now taught as undergraduate course work in most physical therapy programs.

Sherrington's Laws

Several of Sherrington's laws contributed to the development of PNF techniques. His law of reciprocal innervation is particularly important to us because we use it in facilitated stretching. **Reciprocal innervation** (reciprocal inhibition) is a reflex loop mediated by the muscle spindle cells. (Refer to the glossary for definitions of terms that appear in boldface type throughout this book.) When a muscle contracts, reciprocal innervation simultaneously inhibits the opposing muscle. This allows movement to occur around a joint. For instance, when the quadriceps muscle contracts, the hamstring is reciprocally inhibited, thereby allowing the knee to straighten (figure 1.1).

In facilitated stretching, we use reciprocal innervation to maximize the lengthening of the target muscle.

Spiral-Diagonal Patterns

Kabat's research and experimentation led him to realize that movement naturally occurs in spiral-diagonal patterns. The motions required when you comb your hair, swing a golf club, or kick a ball all have spiral (rotational) and diagonal components; that is, they occur not in straight lines but through several planes of motion. If you look at figure 1.2, you can see that the bowler's right arm is moving not only forward but also diagonally up and across his body. You'll also see the spiral component of his motion if you look at the **rotation** of his arm. Spiral-diagonal motion is also taking place in his left arm and right leg.

Even when you walk, your arms naturally move forward and slightly across your body, otherwise your motion would be stiff and robotlike.

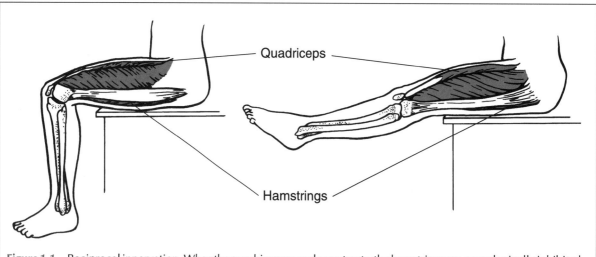

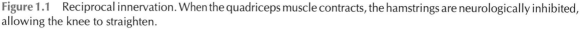

Figure 1.1   Reciprocal innervation. When the quadriceps muscle contracts, the hamstrings are neurologically inhibited, allowing the knee to straighten.

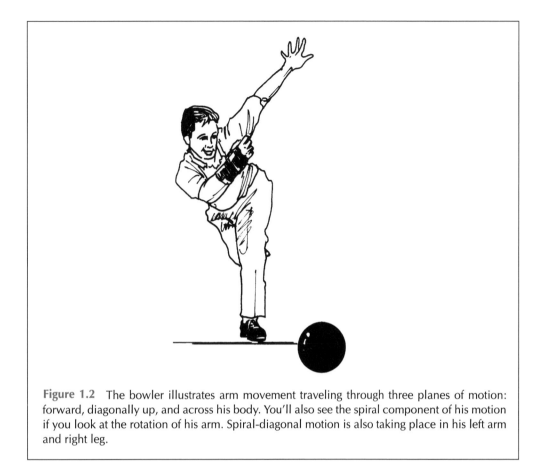

Figure 1.2   The bowler illustrates arm movement traveling through three planes of motion: forward, diagonally up, and across his body. You'll also see the spiral component of his motion if you look at the rotation of his arm. Spiral-diagonal motion is also taking place in his left arm and right leg.

Development of PNF Stretching

In the late 1970s, physical therapists and athletic trainers began using PNF techniques to facilitate flexibility in healthy people. Practitioners began experimenting with variations of the standard techniques, adapting them to their own needs. Some of the terminology changed and versions of PNF stretching became known as "scientific stretching for sport" (3-S technique), "NF technique," "modified PNF," and "facilitated stretching." As word of the effectiveness of these techniques spread, other sport practitioners, including massage therapists, coaches, and sport physicians, began using these techniques.

The rapid growth in sports medicine has fueled the search by practitioners and athletes for effective, efficient techniques for improving performance. The adaptation of PNF stretching techniques for use with athletes opened the door for their current popularity among sports health practitioners, coaches, and the athletes themselves. The use of these techniques will continue to expand as the general public begins to realize the rapid gains in flexibility that are possible.

The Neurophysiological Basis for Facilitated Stretching

Facilitated stretching is based on several neurophysiological mechanisms in the body. A review of these mechanisms will provide the basic understanding you need to perform the techniques properly. Having a good grasp of these theoretical underpinnings will also help you to improvise new stretches not covered in this book.

Muscle Contractions

Two types of muscle contractions, isotonic and isometric, are used in applying the PNF principles. A voluntary contraction that causes movement to occur is called **isotonic contraction.** There are two types of isotonic contractions: **concentric contraction,** in which the muscle shortens as it works, and **eccentric contraction,** in which the muscle resists while being lengthened by an outside force. For example, a concentric isotonic contraction of the pectoral muscles happens when you bring your hands up into the prayer position (figure 1.3). An eccentric contraction of the pectorals would occur if someone else pulls your hands apart while you resist the motion. An eccentric contraction is also called *negative work.*

An **isometric contraction** is a voluntary contraction in which no movement occurs and the muscle length remains unchanged. If you place your hands in the prayer position, and then push, the push isometrically contracts the pectoral muscles.

Stretch Reflexes

A reflex is an automatic, involuntary response to a stimulus. A **stretch reflex** is initiated in response to stretch and helps protect muscles and joints from injury because of overstretching or excessive strain.

The **myotatic stretch reflex** prevents a muscle from stretching too far, too fast, which helps protect the joint from injury. This reflex is commonly seen when a physician is testing your reflexes. She strikes your biceps tendon with a small rubber hammer, and your arm automatically bends at the elbow. Proprioceptors in the biceps, called "muscle spindle cells," monitor the length and tension of the muscle (figure 1.4a). When the muscle lengthens too quickly, as happens when the reflex hammer strikes the tendon, the spindle cells are stimulated and reflexively

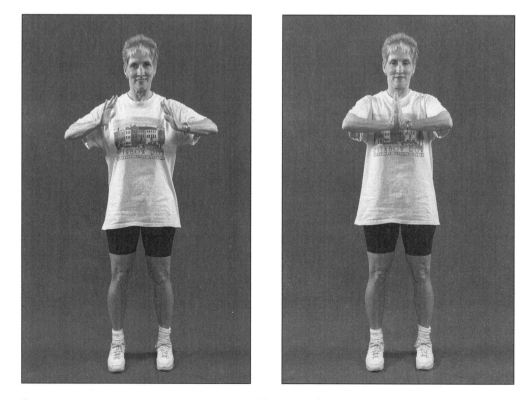

Figure 1.3 A concentric isotonic contraction of the pectoral muscles.

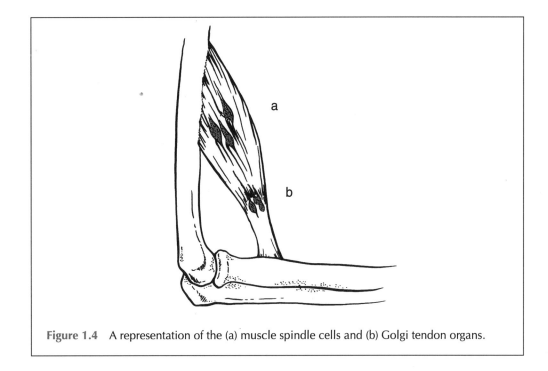

Figure 1.4 A representation of the (a) muscle spindle cells and (b) Golgi tendon organs.

cause the muscle to contract, which causes the arm to bend. This reflexive contraction, the stretch reflex, prevents overstretching of the elbow joint and the biceps.

Because the stretch reflex causes a muscle to contract, we must be careful not to stimulate it during stretching procedures. In performing facilitated stretching, the stretcher actively lengthens the target muscle only to the "stretch barrier" and no farther, thus preventing the stretch reflex from occurring.

The **inverse stretch reflex** (also called autogenic inhibition) has the opposite effect of the myotatic stretch reflex. When the inverse stretch reflex occurs, the muscle relaxes. This reflex is mediated by stretch receptors called Golgi tendon organs (GTOs), which are located in the musculotendinous junction and the tendon. The GTOs monitor the load on the tendon (figure 1.4b). If the load becomes too great, the GTOs are stimulated. They, in turn, cause the muscle to relax through neurological inhibition.

Tendon loading can result from a stretch or a strong contraction, especially an isometric contraction, of the muscle. When a muscle stretch is held, the pull on the tendons should stimulate the GTOs and cause the muscle to relax and lengthen, reducing the chances of muscle tearing. This response is described by Anderson (1984) as the "developmental stretch." He recommends stretching gently, then holding the stretch until the muscle relaxes, allowing you to stretch a little farther. You then hold this new position until the muscle relaxes again, allowing a farther stretch.

Loading also occurs in the tendon when the muscle contracts and pulls on it. Theoretically, when a maximal contraction is elicited from a muscle, the inverse stretch reflex, mediated by the GTOs, should cause the muscle to relax. This is a protective reflex to prevent the muscle and/or the joint from being injured.

Postisometric relaxation (PIR) is another way of describing the inverse stretch reflex that results from a strong isometric contraction. Chaitow, in his text on muscle energy techniques, describes the use of PIR as follows: "Following on from an isometric contraction . . . there is a refractory, or latency, period of approximately 15 seconds during which there can be an easier (due to reduced tone) movement towards the new position (new resistance barrier) of a joint or muscle" (Chaitow 1996, p5).

In facilitated stretching, we use a strong isometric contraction of the target muscle to stimulate the inverse stretch reflex, which relaxes the target muscle and increases its ablity to lengthen.

Chapter 2

Stretching Basics

In this chapter, we look at some of the basic principles and different types of stretching, with a detailed look at facilitated stretching. We also discuss safety issues and proper biomechanics for performing facilitated stretching.

The Stretching Debate

Is stretching necessary? Despite years of research, there is still no clear agreement among the experts on whether stretching is worth the time and effort. However, we can find a consensus that favors daily stretching, especially in conjunction with exercise. In the best of all possible exercise schemes, the athlete warms up, stretches, exercises, stretches again, and then cools down.

For years, the debate about stretching has been based on whether there were any tangible benefits. Proponents of stretching claim that it helps prevent injuries, prevents soreness, improves performance, promotes body awareness, stimulates blood flow, and is mentally relaxing and centering. Opponents argue that stretching is a waste of time, can actually cause injury, and does nothing to improve performance or prevent soreness or injuries. Each side has a multitude of studies, reports, and anecdotal evidence to support its claims.

Common Ground

The physiological evidence is clear, however. When you stretch, it's more effective if the muscles are already warmed up. A warm-up entails light activity, similar to what your exercise will be, for 10 to 15 minutes. This activity increases blood flow to the muscles you'll be using and gets them ready to work. Warming up also helps to reduce stiffness, making the muscles more supple. I like to use the example of taffy, which is stiff and brittle when it's cold. When you warm it up, it becomes more pliable and stretches easily. Think of your muscles in the same way. As the muscle fibers warm up, they become more pliable and supple, and stretch more easily.

Grant discusses other benefits of warming up, including increased production of synovial fluid to lubricate joints, increased oxygen exchange in the muscle, increased rate of nerve transmission, and more efficient cooperation of the muscles around a joint (1997). If you warm up first, your stretching exercises will be more effective and efficient, you'll make greater gains than if you're stretching cold, and you'll be less likely to injure yourself.

In the ideal world, we'd stretch after warming up, exercise, then stretch again after exercise as part of the cooldown process. The reasoning behind stretching twice goes like this:

1. Stretch the muscles before a workout to get them ready to perform at their optimum length. This optimum length allows the muscles to develop the most power as they work.

2. Stretch the muscles after exercise while they're still warm to bring them back to their optimum resting length. As muscles work they repeatedly contract and shorten, and they tend to stay short when the workout is over unless you stretch them again. Postexercise stretching can be incorporated into the cooldown.

If time is a factor (and when isn't it these days), we recommend skipping the preexercise stretching and concentrating on postexercise stretching. If you don't stretch before exercise, be sure to complete a thorough warm-up before getting into your main workout. Postexercise stretching will return those tired muscles to their normal resting length as you go about the rest of your daily activities. In postexercise stretching, there is some danger of overstretching the muscles because they may be too pliable. But if done with awareness the risk is minimal and is far outweighed by the benefits gained.

Pain-Free Stretching

Many people stretch incorrectly, believing that it must hurt to be effective. Our belief is that stretching must be completely comfortable to be effective. If the muscle you are attempting to stretch hurts, the body's natural response will be to tighten up to prevent any more lengthening, and possible injury, to that muscle. We advocate taking the muscle to its "soft tissue barrier," which means the point at which you begin to feel some resistance to further stretching. The soft tissue barrier is the starting point for the stretch.

Pain-free stretching also applies to the rest of the body during a specific stretch. If the stretcher is in an uncomfortable position, even though there is no pain in the target muscle, we don't believe he will be able to get the best results from the stretch. For example, if the stretcher experiences low back pain during the quadriceps stretch, he won't be able to relax and fully engage in the process. Repositioning the stretcher to relieve the low back discomfort makes the quadriceps stretch more effective.

Types of Stretching

Many types of stretching are in use today, some of which are variations developed for specific sports or activities. Stretching can be broadly categorized as passive, active, or some blend of the two. These categories can be further subdivided into two types of stretching: ballistic and static.

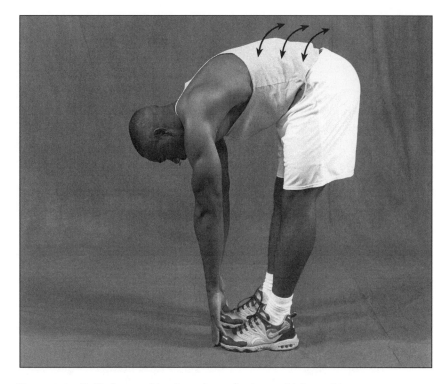

Figure 2.1   Ballistic stretching is performed using rapid, bouncing movements.

Ballistic and Static Stretching

Ballistic, or *dynamic, stretching* is done using rapid, bouncing movements to force the target muscle to elongate (figure 2.1). This can be done actively or passively. This type of stretching is generally out of favor because it may elicit a strong myotatic stretch reflex and leave the muscle shorter than its prestretching length. Beaulieu (1981) asserts that ballistic stretching creates more than twice the tension in the target muscle, compared with a static stretch. This increases the likelihood of tearing the muscle because the rapid bouncing does not allow enough time for the inverse stretch reflex to be engaged and for the muscle to relax.

Static stretching has been popularized by Bob Anderson in his book, *Stretching* (1984). The muscle to be stretched (target muscle) is lengthened slowly (to inhibit firing of the stretch reflex) and held in a comfortable range for 15 to 30 seconds. As the position is held, the feeling of stretch diminishes (possibly because of the inverse stretch reflex), and the stretcher moves gently into a deeper stretch and holds again (figure 2.2). Static stretching can be done actively or passively.

Passive and Active Stretching

Passive stretching is done to the stretcher by a partner; it can be ballistic or static. The stretcher relaxes and the partner moves the limb being stretched to gain new **range of motion** (ROM) (figure 2.3). Passive stretching is often used to increase flexibility at the extremes of range of motion, as in gymnastics, where maximum flexibility is crucial for performance. It is also used when active movement is painful.

Done carelessly or with poor form, passive stretching can cause muscle injury. It is risky because the person assisting the stretching cannot feel the sensations of the stretcher and may overstretch the muscle. Passive stretching requires good communication between the stretcher and the partner.

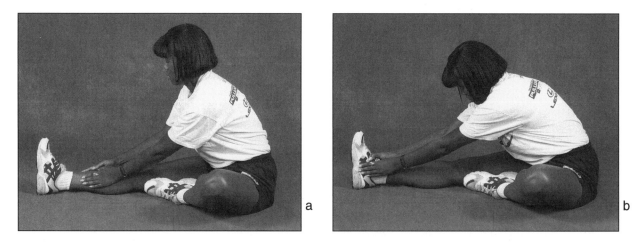

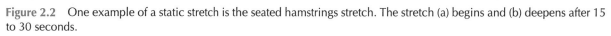

Figure 2.2 One example of a static stretch is the seated hamstrings stretch. The stretch (a) begins and (b) deepens after 15 to 30 seconds.

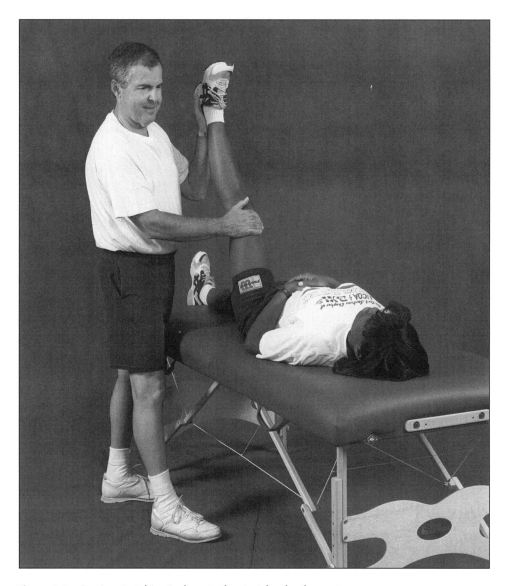

Figure 2.3 Passive stretching is done to the stretcher by the partner.

Active stretching means that the stretcher is doing the work instead of having a partner do it. Active forms of stretching are generally considered safer than passive stretching because the chance of overstretching and causing injury are greatly reduced when the stretcher controls the force and duration of the stretch.

Active-assisted stretching combines active movement by the stretcher with help from a partner, either to add passive stretch or to provide resistance to motion, thus blending active and passive stretching types.

Muscle Energy Technique (MET)

Another form of active-assisted stretching is the muscle energy technique (MET), an osteopathic technique that evolved from PNF. According to Chaitow, MET "targets the soft tissues primarily, although it also makes a major contribution towards joint mobilization . . . " (Chaitow 1996, p1). Like PNF techniques, MET uses an isometric contraction of the target muscle before the stretch. MET, however, uses only minimal force during the isometric phase. The stretching phase is generally, though not always, done passively. Because MET developed in osteopathic medicine, it has the further goal of joint mobilization, which is not a goal of PNF techniques.

Some variations/refinements of MET include the following:

• *The Lewit Technique (PIR)*—Dr. Karel Lewit, a Czech neurologist, refers to his method as PIR, which stands for postisometric relaxation. The name refers to the neurological inhibition of a muscle following its isometric contraction.

• *Reciprocal Inhibition (RI)*—You'll recall from our discussion in chapter 1 that reciprocal inhibition describes a neurological reflex that causes one muscle to relax when its opposing muscle contracts. RI is used to stretch a target muscle by first contracting the opposing muscle. This contraction inhibits the target muscle and allows it to be stretched farther. RI is often used by sports massage therapists as a technique to relieve muscle cramps in athletes after strenuous competition. The therapist will have the athlete isometrically contract the muscle opposite the one which is cramping, thereby inhibiting the cramping muscle, which then relaxes.

Active Isolated Stretching

Active isolated stretching (AIS) was developed by Aaron Mattes and is detailed in his book by the same name (Mattes 1995). AIS uses active movement and reciprocal inhibition, but not isometric work, to achieve greater flexibility. AIS can also be performed with a partner as an active-assisted technique. Mattes recommends isolating the muscle to be stretched, then actively lengthening it to a point of "light irritation." Hold this position for no more than two seconds, then return the limb to the starting position. This sequence is usually repeated 8 to 10 times. This stretching protocol is thought to prevent the stretch reflex, while activating reciprocal inhibition, thereby allowing the target muscle to lengthen more easily.

PNF Stretching

Facilitated stretching is based on the principles of PNF and is one of several variations of PNF stretching. Some of the other versions of PNF stretching are referred to as modified PNF (Moore and Hutton 1980; Cornelius and Craft-Hamm 1988), NF (Surburg 1981), and scientific stretching for sports (3-S technique; Holt 1976).

Most PNF stretching techniques are done passively or as active-assisted exercises. The two main types of PNF stretching, also called relaxation techniques by Voss (1985), are *hold-relax* and *contract-relax*.

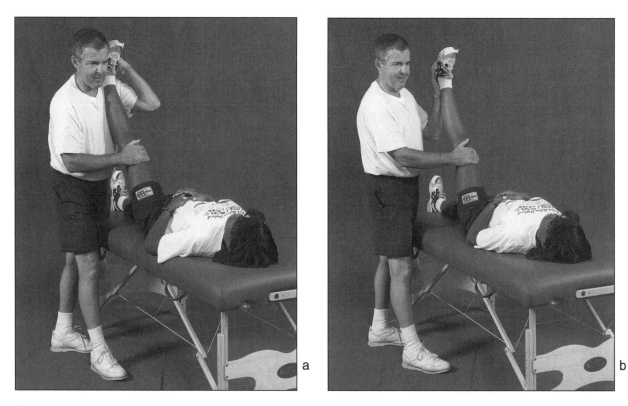

Figure 2.4 The PNF hold-relax hamstrings stretch. (a) The stretcher isometrically contracts her hamstrings to resist the partner's attempt to move her leg into flexion. (b) The stretcher actively moves into a deeper stretch.

Hold-relax (HR) is generally used if range of motion is extremely limited or if active movement is not available because of weakness and/or pain. The stretcher holds the limb at its lengthened range of motion and isometrically resists the therapist's attempt to move the limb into a deeper stretch of the target muscle. The stretcher then relaxes and actively moves the limb into the new range (figure 2.4).

Contract-relax (CR) is also used with marked limitation in range of motion. This technique combines isotonic and isometric work. Using CR, the physical therapist moves the limb passively to the point of limitation, then instructs the patient to try to move the limb into the shortened range. The physical therapist resists but allows rotation of the limb. All other effort by the patient is isometric. The therapist then moves the limb passively into a new range of motion. After several rounds of CR, the patient is instructed to move actively through the new range of motion.

Facilitated Stretching Sequence: Simplified Version

Facilitated stretching is active-assisted stretching, which uses active motion and isometric work to improve flexibility and enhance motor learning in the process. Simplified, the three steps involved in facilitated stretching are:

1. actively lengthen the target muscle,
2. isometrically contract the target muscle, and
3. actively lengthen the target muscle again.

Facilitated stretching is also called CRAC, an acronym for contract relax antagonist contract. CRAC is a modified form of PNF stretching in which the stretcher performs all the work, and you act only as facilitator. For example, during the

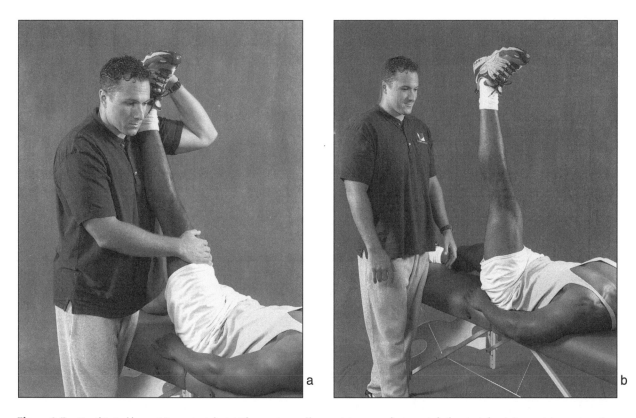

Figure 2.5 Facilitated hamstrings stretch. (a) The partner offers resistance only to match the stretcher's isometric contraction of the hamstrings. (b) The stretcher actively moves into a deeper stretch with no help from the partner. Here, the partner has removed his hands from the stretcher to illustrate the stretcher's active movement. In an actual stretch, the partner maintains the stretcher's knee in extension.

hamstrings stretch, the stretcher begins by actively moving his leg to the starting position, then isometrically contracts, then relaxes his hamstring as you provide resistance. Then, through an antagonist contraction of the quadriceps and psoas (hip flexors) to lift the leg higher, the stretcher actively lengthens the hamstrings (figure 2.5).

In the available research that included CRAC techniques, CRAC stretching was found to be the most effective in achieving gains in range of motion (Moore and Hutton 1980; Cornelius 1983; Etnyre and Abraham 1986a).

Safety Issues

Facilitated stretches (CRAC) entail virtually no risk of injury because there is no passive movement involved—the stretcher does all the work. You act only as a facilitator for the technique and make no attempt to increase the stretch. This factor addresses the concern of some investigators that poorly trained or inattentive partners could cause injury by being too vigorous in moving the limb to a new range of motion (Beaulieu 1981; Surburg 1983).

Philosophy

In addition to the effectiveness and safety issues addressed previously, there is also a philosophical basis for using facilitated stretching over other styles. We want to avoid making the stretcher dependent on us, and we want to encourage his own body awareness. With facilitated stretching, the stretcher learns to do it for himself and becomes more body aware in the process.

It's very easy for the stretcher to become dependent on a partner, and passive forms of stretching, in which the partner does it to or for the stretcher, encourage this passive mind-set. Facilitated stretching is designed to be done by the stretcher, and the partner acts only as a facilitator. Self-stretching is emphasized so that the stretcher can do it alone, using some easy-to-find accessories to replace the partner. This places responsibility for success squarely where it belongs, with the stretcher.

Facilitated stretching is designed to improve the communication between and among the muscles and the nervous system. The muscles only do what they are told to do by the nervous system. Therefore, their interaction must be clear. By actively engaging the muscles throughout the routine, learning takes place that allows the muscles to work more efficiently. The muscle spindle cells and the Golgi tendon organs are stimulated, reciprocal inhibition reflexes are strengthened, and the muscles learn to work better together. In passive work, this does not occur because an outside force is at work, which requires little neurological or muscular involvement from the stretcher. The two main neurological effects we see from facilitated stretching are as follows:

• *Postisometric Relaxation (PIR)*. It appears that a muscle is more relaxed and able to lengthen after a strong isometric contraction. This readiness to lengthen may be the result of the inverse stretch reflex, which is mediated by the Golgi tendon organs. We use this physiological response to prepare the muscle to stretch.

• *Reciprocal Inhibition*. When one muscle contracts, the opposing muscle relaxes because of neurological inhibition, thereby allowing movement to occur around a joint. This reflex is mediated by the muscle spindle cells. We use this inhibition loop to actively lengthen the target muscle.

Facilitated Stretching Sequence: Detailed Version

As mentioned earlier, facilitated stretching is best done with a partner, although many of the stretches can be done alone, assisted by accessories. The more detailed steps involved in a partner-assisted facilitated stretch are as follows:

1. The stretcher actively lengthens the muscle to be stretched (the target muscle) to its maximal pain-free end range. This is also called the soft tissue barrier or stretch barrier. This active movement incorporates reciprocal inhibition (figure 2.6).

For example, if you wish to stretch the hamstring, have the stretcher lie on his back and contract his quadriceps and psoas (hip flexors) to actively lift the leg as high as possible, keeping the knee straight. You may need to hold the knee straight as the stretcher lifts his leg. This stretches the hamstrings to their end range. As the hip flexors contract to lift the leg, the hamstrings are reciprocally inhibited.

2. As the partner, you then position yourself to offer resistance for the stretcher to isometrically contract the target muscle against. For stretching the hamstring, support the lower leg against your shoulder or by holding it with both hands.

3. Direct the stretcher to begin *slowly* and "push" or "pull" to isometrically contract the target muscle as you provide matching resistance. Don't allow the stretcher to overpower you. When the stretcher has achieved the proper level of isometric contraction, hold it for 6 to 10 seconds. This isometric contraction stimulates the Golgi tendon organs, and this stimulation causes postisometric relaxation.

4. The stretcher then relaxes the isometric contraction and inhales deeply. During this time, maintain the limb in the starting position.

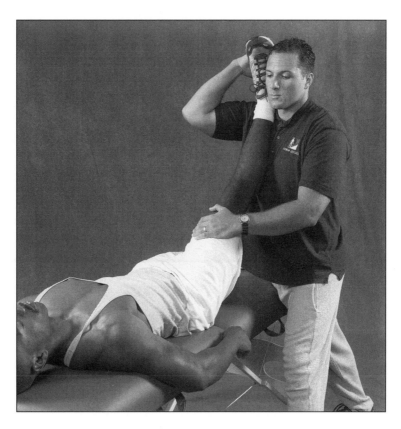

Figure 2.6   Starting position of the hamstrings stretch (right leg). Support the stretcher's leg using proper biomechanics.

5.   On the exhale, the stretcher contracts the antagonist (the opposing muscle—in this case the quads and psoas) and pulls the target muscle into a deeper stretch, once again using reciprocal inhibition to enhance the stretch (figure 2.7). As the partner, you should never push or pull to deepen the stretch.

6.   Now the partner moves into the new position to once again offer resistance.

7.   Repeat the process 2 to 3 times.

PNF stretches should always be pain free. If the stretcher experiences pain, try repositioning the limb or use less force during the isometric contraction of the target muscle. If pain persists, don't use PNF for that particular muscle until you've determined why it's causing pain.

Use of Language: Push/Pull Versus Resist

In general, your instruction to the stretcher will be to either "push" or "pull" during the isometric phase. This communicates more clearly what you wish to have happen. If you ask the stretcher to "resist," you are communicating that you will be doing something to her that she needs to act against. In fact, you want her to contract the muscle, the force of which you, as the facilitator, will resist. This also refers back to our discussion of empowering the stretcher to take an active, rather than passive, role in the process.

Breathing

Muscles need oxygen to work. But many times, we are in the habit of holding our breath during strong muscular effort. How do we reconcile these two conflicting

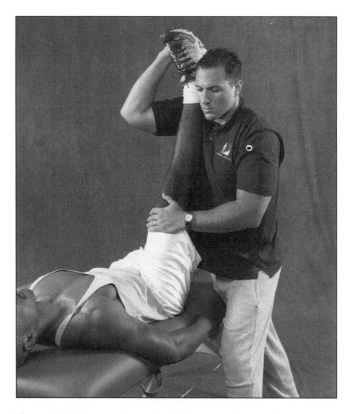

Figure 2.7 The stretcher actively deepens the stretch.

facts? I think it's more important to breathe, especially because we are not asking for maximal effort on the part of the stretcher during any part of the sequence. Another reason for normal breathing is that holding the breath during the isometric phase is often accompanied by compensatory recruitment of other muscles. And third, there is some risk that holding the breath during muscular contraction may raise the blood pressure.

It's easy to monitor the stretcher's breathing and your own throughout the process. We've found that three cycles of normal breathing (in and out) takes about 6 to 10 seconds, which is the length of time we want for the isometric contraction.

Safety Issues

Stretching safely is of utmost concern for both the stretcher and the partner. Body mechanics are extremely important during all phases of stretching, especially during the isometric phase. Plan carefully and communicate freely with each other. The partner applying the resistance may be expending unnecessary energy (because of poor ergonomics), or the stretcher may be working too hard. Not only can you become acutely injured by using these techniques carelessly, but you can develop overuse syndromes unnecessarily.

Safety for the Partner

The athletic stance, which is common to most sports, adheres to the principles of good body mechanics and prepares the athlete for optimum performance. The legs are set wide apart; the knees are usually slightly bent; the back is relatively straight; the head is upright; the center of gravity is evenly distributed; and the use of the powerful leg muscles is stressed. Most people have used this stance at some time in their lives because it is the most prepared position for the body to receive a force. It is the "strongest" position.

When you are acting as the partner during facilitated stretching, you may be at risk for injury if you don't take care of yourself. By paying attention to your posture and body mechanics, you can eliminate the possibility of injury. When you are acting as the partner in facilitated stretching, be sure to maintain an athletic stance.

Some areas of the athletic stance to pay attention to include the following:

• As you work, pay attention to your legs and feet. Use a wide stance to help you remain balanced and stable, especially as you resist the isometric contraction of the stretcher.

• Be aware of keeping your spine lengthened as you work, instead of collapsing into yourself. This lengthening helps prevent undue stress on the spine.

• Keep your low back area flattened to reduce pressure on your lumbar spine. This will help prevent low back pain. Tighten your abdominal muscles to help keep your back from arching too far.

• Remember that you control the strength of the stretcher's isometric contraction. Provide resistance only up to the level that is comfortable for you, then ask the stretcher to hold at that level of effort.

• Avoid unnecessary twisting or bending. Instead, have the stretcher move to accommodate you.

• Use the large muscles of the trunk and extremities to resist the isometric contraction instead of smaller, weaker muscles. For instance, have the stretcher push against your shoulder rather than your arm during a hamstrings stretch.

• To avoid losing your balance when you're acting as the partner, you control the session and give the commands so that you're prepared to resist the isometric contraction. Be sure that the stretcher begins slowly during the isometric phase.

• Stop immediately if either person has pain, discuss it to determine the cause, and correct the problem before continuing.

Safety for the Stretcher

Because the stretcher does most of the work in facilitated stretching, it's common to see compensation patterns at work, especially during the isometric phase. For this reason, we need to pay attention to the stretcher's mechanics and stabilization.

When I first started doing facilitated stretching, I was taught to stabilize the stretcher when necessary to prevent compensatory shifts in position, which recruit muscles inappropriately or unnecessarily. Over the years, I've come to realize that the stretcher needs to take an active role in preventing compensation. The active learning translates into his daily life. If he can learn to use his gluteus maximus and hamstrings without compensation on the table, then he'll be more likely to carry that new, correct behavior into his everyday activities.

Another component of having the stretcher more involved in stabilizing his motion is the discovery of where he is unaware. For instance, in attempting to stretch the quadratus lumborum, many people are unable to isolate the muscle. They begin recruiting like mad to try to do the simple motion required for the stretch. This discovery enables us to work together to figure out how to simply contract this quadratus lumborum without bringing in other muscles inappropriately. The learning that results is extremely useful for the stretcher as he incorporates it into his "real" life.

Importance of Positioning   To achieve the most benefit from stretching, our goal is to position the stretcher to isolate the target muscle as much as possible. This isolation ensures that the target muscle is the primary one contracting during the isometric phase and being stretched during the lengthening phase. Although it's impossible to completely isolate and activate only one muscle, careless positioning allows inappropriate, compensatory muscle recruitment and interferes with achieving optimum results from facilitated stretching.

Compensation Patterns We all develop compensatory patterns of muscular contraction to make up for muscle weakness or imbalance, postural distortions, structural irregularities, and the like. When performing facilitated stretching, many of these patterns of compensation become obvious. For instance, when doing a hamstring stretch, we very often see the hip lift off the table when the stretcher is isometrically contracting the hamstring. This unconscious shift engages the gluteus maximus more and is usually because of a weak hamstring.

By being aware of compensation and working with the stretcher to eliminate it during facilitated stretching, we'll achieve better results on the table and the stretcher will learn to move more efficiently as she goes about her daily life. Where appropriate, we've indicated the common compensation patterns associated with a stretch.

Reducing Fatigue

Because facilitated stretching is an active form of work, it can be fatiguing for both the stretcher and the partner. Reducing fatigue can reduce the chance of injury.

For the stretcher, it's important to remember that maximal effort is not necessary. We need only a good contraction of the target muscle during the isometric phase. This can be especially important for stretchers who don't participate in a regular exercise program because they may experience delayed onset muscle soreness the day after a stretching session if they work too hard.

For you, the partner, reducing fatigue becomes an issue if you are working with several people throughout the day. Injuries are more likely if you're fatigued. One of the benefits of facilitated stretching is that the stretcher does most of the work. As the partner, your main task is to assist the stretcher, not do the work for her. The stretcher moves the limb into position; you don't have to lift it or support it for her except for brief periods during the sequence. Relax whenever possible during the session and expend only the effort necessary.

If you're using good body mechanics, you will usually have a mechanical advantage when resisting the isometric contraction of the stretcher. This leverage allows you to accomplish your work with minimal physical effort.

Self-Stretching Principles

In keeping with the theme of stretcher learning and self-help, our goal is to teach the stretcher to incorporate facilitated stretching into his daily routine without the need to rely on a partner. For this reason, most of the stretches presented here will include a self-stretch version. The principles for self-stretching are just like the ones for partner work:

- Use proper positioning to isolate the target muscle.
- Use self-stabilization to prevent compensation.
- Breathe correctly.
- Assert appropriate effort during isometric phase.
- Stretch the target muscle by contracting the antagonist.
- Remain pain free throughout the sequence.

Chapter 3

Spiral-Diagonal Patterns

The spiral is an inescapable component of life. I'm indebted to Thomas Hendrickson, DC, for permission to quote at length from his book, *Manual of Orthopedic Massage.*

We live in a spiral universe. Our local galaxy, the Milky Way, forms a spiral. The spiral is a fundamental shape in the movement of air currents over the surface of the Earth. Water, which covers 71% of the Earth's surface, moves in a spiral pattern not only as it snakes its way across the land, but also as it spirals internally in the form of secondary currents within the moving water.

The spiral is also an essential pattern in the body. Like the Earth, the human body is about 70% water. The blood within the arteries moves in a spiral pattern. Muscles are also organized in spirals, both macroscopically and microscopically. The levator scapula, for example, makes a spiral turn from its attachments on the scapula to the cervical spine.

Microscopically, actin and myosin are the two basic proteins that compose muscle fiber. Each actin filament is a double helix, composed of two strands that spiral around each other. And myosin contains globular heads that spiral around the myosin filament. The gross structure of the tendon and ligament is also a spiral. Tendons, ligaments, and bones are composed mostly of Type I collagen, which is a triple helix. On the macroscopic level, the long bones, such as the humerus, spiral along their axes. And DNA, the smallest structure in the physical body, is a triple helix. (Hendrickson 1995, p3)

Rationale and Development of Spiral Patterns

PNF is based on spiral-diagonal movement. Kabat, Knott, and Voss noticed that normal movements found in sports and physical activities are spiral-diagonal in nature. They defined these "mass movement patterns" as "various combinations of motion . . . (that) require shortening and lengthening reactions of many muscles in varying degrees" (Voss et al. 1985, p1). The spiral-diagonal character of normal movements arises from the design of the skeletal system and the placement of the muscles on it. The muscles spiral around the bones from origin to insertion, and therefore, when they contract, they tend to create that spiral in motion.

This spiral is especially noticeable in the movements of your arms, which swing across your body as you walk or run. When the biceps contract, they not only flex your elbow, they also rotate (**supinate**) your forearm (figure 3.1a-c). Many muscles are actually capable of motion in three planes. For instance, the psoas muscle flexes the hip (the dominant action) but also assists **adduction** and external rotation of the femur (figure 3.2).

Voss et al. (1985) suggest learning the PNF patterns through free-movement exercises. These give a sense of the natural rhythm of the patterns and let you feel the movements through a full range of motion. Even though we don't use the full patterns in facilitated stretching, learning them will make it easier to visualize the range of motion you're trying to improve as you incorporate them into stretching.

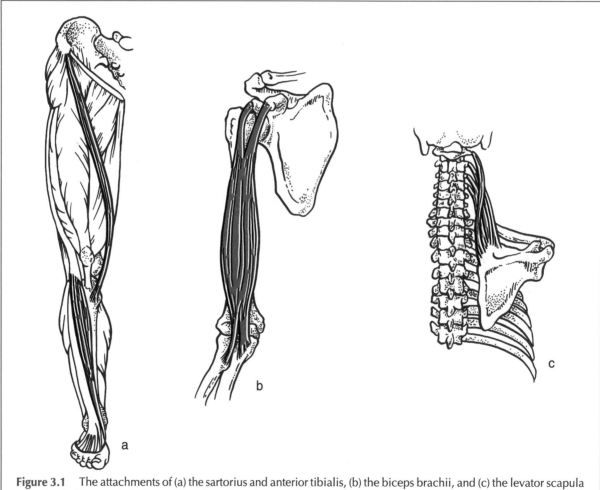

Figure 3.1   The attachments of (a) the sartorius and anterior tibialis, (b) the biceps brachii, and (c) the levator scapula muscles facilitate spiral-diagonal motion when the muscles contract.

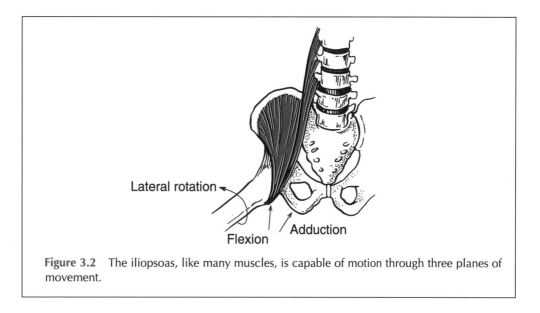

Figure 3.2 The iliopsoas, like many muscles, is capable of motion through three planes of movement.

Patterns for the Arm

There are two basic PNF patterns for the arm: D1 and D2. Each pattern is divided into two parts: **flexion** and **extension.** The movement sequence for the D1 extension pattern is the exact opposite of the sequence for D1 flexion. The same is true for D2 extension and D2 flexion.

D1 Patterns for the Arm

The first pattern is called D1 (D is for diagonal) and is divided into D1 flexion and D1 extension. The patterns are named for their *ending* positions. D1 flexion of the arm *ends* in flexion, adduction, and external rotation, which means it *begins* in the opposite position of extension, **abduction,** and internal rotation (see figure 3.3). D1 extension *ends* in extension, abduction, and internal rotation, so must *begin* in flexion, adduction, and external rotation.

This makes more sense when you perform the pattern instead of just reading about it. So take a moment now and practice D1 before going on.

D1 Practice: Arm

1. Stand and bring your right arm up and across your body, with your arm rotated so that the thumb side of your hand points forward, as in figure 3.3a. Specifically, this is flexion, **horizontal adduction,** and external rotation of the humerus. The right forearm is supinated, and the wrist and fingers are flexed.

2. Go as far in each plane of motion as you can to fully lengthen all the involved muscles. This is the beginning position for D1 extension. It's also the ending position for D1 flexion.

3. From this starting position, slowly move your arm diagonally, down, out, and back to arrive at the same arm and hand position as the model in figure 3.3c. This motion blends internal rotation, abduction, and extension of the humerus, **pronation** of the forearm, and extension of the wrist and fingers. This is the ending position for D1 extension. It's also the starting position for D1 flexion.

4. From this position, retrace your motion to arrive once again at your starting position.

Reverse push-ups →

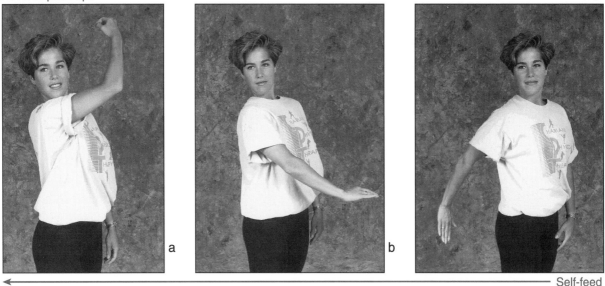

a   b   c

← Self-feed

Figure 3.3   The D1 pattern for the upper extremity. D1 extension (reverse push-ups): (a) initiation, (b) midphase, and (c) end position. D1 flexion (self-feed): (c) initiation, (b) midphase, and (a) end position.

Repeat these patterns several times with each arm, and then with both together, until you feel the rhythm. What activities use motion like this? Throwing a Frisbee, swinging a golf club or a baseball bat, picking up a hat and putting it on your head, working as a grocery checker, and putting food in your mouth all use patterns of movement that have components of the D1 pattern. It may help you remember the ends of each pattern by giving them nicknames. "Reverse push-ups," as in figure 3.3c, put you in D1 extension; you can think of D1 flexion, 3.3a, as the "self-feeding" pattern.

D2 Patterns for the Arm

The second arm pattern, D2, uses the diagonal *opposite* to D1 and is also divided into D2 flexion and D2 extension. D2 flexion *ends* in flexion, abduction, and external rotation, which means it *begins* in extension, adduction, and internal rotation. D2 extension *ends* in extension, adduction, and internal rotation, so must *begin* in flexion, abduction, and external rotation.

Once again, the patterns make more sense when you perform them. So take some time to practice D2 now, before going on.

D2 Practice: Arm

1. Stand and bring your right arm up, out, and slightly behind your body, with your arm rotated so the thumb faces behind you, as in figure 3.4a. This is flexion, abduction, and external rotation of the humerus. The right forearm is supinated, with the wrist and fingers extended.

2. Go as far in each plane of motion as you can to fully lengthen all the involved muscles. This is the beginning position for D2 extension. It's also the ending position for D2 flexion because the patterns are named for their ending positions.

3. From this starting position, slowly move your arm diagonally down and across your body, as if you were putting a sword back into its scabbard, ending up in the same position as the model in figure 3.4c. This motion blends internal rotation, adduction, and extension of the humerus. The forearm pronates, and the wrist and fingers flex. For the sake of practice, you are now at the ending position for D2 extension. In reality, the ending position would be through the body, in a "hammerlock" position, to be sure the

Sheath sword

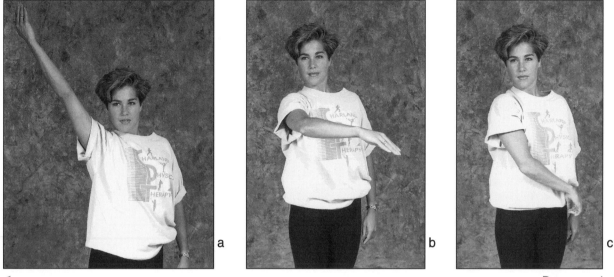

Draw sword

Figure 3.4 The D2 pattern for the upper extremity. D2 extension (sheathing a sword): (a) initiation, (b) midphase, and (c) end position. D2 flexion (drawing a sword): (c) initiation, (b) midphase, and (a) end position.

arm is fully extended and internally rotated. The ending position for D2 extension is also the starting position for D2 flexion.

4. Now, retrace your motion (D2 flexion pattern) to arrive back at your starting point.

Repeat these patterns several times with each arm, and then with both together, until they begin to feel natural and easy. What activities use motion like this? Throwing a ball, drawing a sword, using a hockey stick, lifting and stacking, washing windows, and taking a sweater off over your head all use patterns of movement that have components of the D2 pattern. It may help you remember the ends of each pattern by giving them nicknames. We'll call D2 extension "sheathing a sword" and D2 flexion "drawing a sword."

Patterns for the Leg

When you feel competent with the arm patterns, you can move on to the legs. As with the arm, there are two patterns for the leg: D1 and D2. Once again, each pattern is divided into two parts: flexion and extension. The patterns are similar but not identical.

D1 Patterns for the Leg

The D1 diagonal for the leg is divided into D1 flexion and D1 extension. D1 flexion *ends* in flexion, adduction, and external rotation of the leg, so must *begin* in extension, abduction, and internal rotation. D1 extension *ends* in extension, abduction, and internal rotation, so *begins* in flexion, adduction, and external rotation.

Active practice will make this easier to understand.

D1 Practice: Leg

You'll find it easier to do this practice if you use a wall or a chair for balance and support.

1. Stand and bring your right leg forward and across your body, rotating the leg so your foot points to the right. This is flexion, adduction, and external rotation of the femur, **dorsiflexion** and **inversion** of the foot, and extension of the toes.

Toe-off ───►

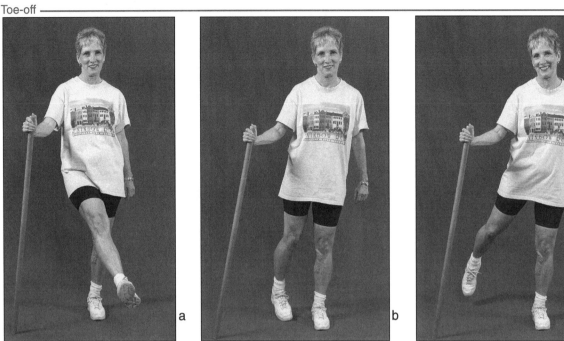

a   b   c

◄─────────────────────────────────────── Soccer kick

Figure 3.5   The D1 pattern for the lower extremity. D1 extension (toe-off): (a) initiation, (b) midphase, and (c) end position. D1 flexion (soccer kick): (c) initiation, (b) midphase, and (a) end position.

2. Go as far in each plane of motion as you can to fully lengthen all the involved muscles. This is the beginning position for D1 extension. It's also the ending position for D1 flexion. Check your position against the model in figure 3.5a.

3. Slowly swing your leg, beginning with internal rotation, to end up with the leg behind and away from your body, with the foot pointing to the left. This is extension, abduction, and internal rotation of the femur, **plantarflexion** and **eversion** of the foot, and flexion of the toes. Compare your position with that of the model in figure 3.5c. This is the ending position for D1 extension. It's also the starting position for D1 flexion.

4. From this position, retrace your motion to arrive once again where you started.

Swing your leg through this pattern several times to feel the rhythm of it. Many athletic activities require aspects of the D1 pattern. Dancers, skaters, and soccer players, to name a few, all need coordination and flexibility through the D1 pattern. D1 flexion is called the "soccer kick." You can remember D1 extension as "toe-off."

D2 Patterns for the Leg

The second pattern for the leg, D2, uses the diagonal *opposite* to D1 and is also divided into D2 flexion and D2 extension. D2 flexion *ends* in flexion, abduction, and internal rotation of the leg, which means it *begins* in extension, adduction, and external rotation. D2 extension *begins* in flexion, abduction, and internal rotation and *ends* in extension, adduction, and external rotation.

Active practice makes it clearer.

D2 Practice: Leg

1. Stand and bring your right leg forward and out away from your body, rotating the leg so your foot points to the left. This is flexion, abduction, and internal rotation. The foot is dorsiflexed and everted, and the toes are extended.

Turnout

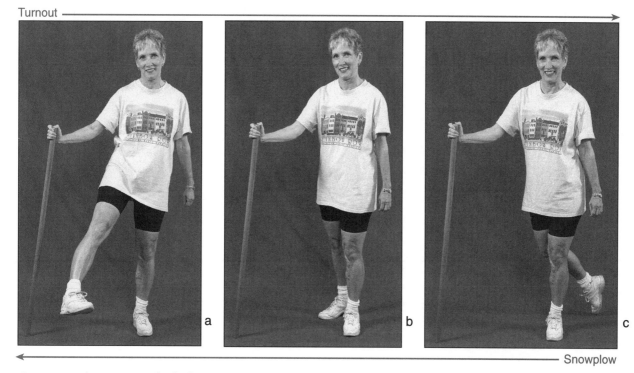

Snowplow

Figure 3.6   The D2 pattern for the lower extremity. D2 extension (turnout): (a) initiation, (b) midphase, and (c) end position. D2 flexion (snowplow): (c) initiation, (b) midphase, and (a) end position.

2. Go as far in each plane of motion as you can to fully lengthen all the involved muscles. This is the beginning position for D2 extension and the ending position for D2 flexion. Compare your position to the model in figure 3.6a.

3. Slowly swing your leg back and across your body, rotating the leg externally. This is extension, adduction, and external rotation of the femur. The foot is plantarflexed and inverted, and the toes are flexed.

4. Go as far in each plane of motion as you can to fully lengthen all the involved muscles. You've achieved the end of D2 extension and the beginning of D2 flexion. Check your position with the model in figure 3.6c.

As you practice this D2 pattern a few times, does it remind you of any activity? If you're a skier, you may recognize components of the snowplow turn in D2 flexion. To help you remember it, we'll call D2 flexion the "snowplow." D2 extension reminds some people of a ballet position, so we'll call D2 extension "turnout."

Using the Patterns for Stretching

The full spiral-diagonal patterns use movement through three planes of motion: extension or flexion, adduction or abduction, and rotation. When a physical therapist uses these PNF patterns with a patient, the goal is to restore or increase strength and coordination, as well as to increase range of motion.

In facilitated stretching, our primary goal is to increase range of motion quickly and efficiently. We stretch groups of related muscles simultaneously when we use these three-dimensional patterns, thereby gaining greater benefit in a shorter amount of time.

Working at the End of Range

For stretching, we employ only the lengthened position of the pattern, preventing the limb from going through its range of motion. The stretcher assumes the starting

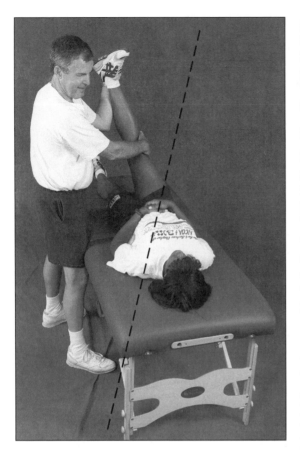

Figure 3.7   Visualize a diagonal line through opposite corners of the table. Use this line as a guide for the movement of the leg to be sure you have a balanced blend of flexion and adduction.

position of the pattern (lengthened range), but her attempts to move the limb through the pattern are isometric; that is, she pushes or pulls in all three planes of motion, but we allow no movement to occur. The stretch occurs when the stretcher actively moves farther into the lengthened range of the pattern.

Rotational Component

In the first edition of *Facilitated Stretching*, we recommended allowing rotation and isometrically resisting the other two directions of the pattern. This was based on our understanding of statements made by Voss et al. (1985). Subsequent reading, discussion with other experts, and our own experience has convinced us that, for our purposes, the rotational component of the pattern can also be isometric without any loss of results. This change also makes it less complicated to perform the stretch.

Blending Adduction/Flexion or Abduction/Extension

When we're using the patterns, our goal is to emphasize the diagonal line of stretch. For instance, in the D1 pattern, we don't want too much adduction, or too much flexion, but a blend of both. It may be helpful to visualize a diagonal line through opposite corners of the table or plinth on which the stretcher is lying (figure 3.7). You can use this diagonal line as a guide for the movement of the arm or leg to be sure you have a balanced blend of adduction/flexion or abduction/extension.

Although this blend of motion is usually what we're looking for, there may be times when you wish to emphasize one over the other. For instance, you may find that the stretcher's motion is more limited in adduction than flexion. You can improve her range in adduction by deviating from the diagonal to emphasize more adduction and less flexion.

Neurological Benefit of Precise Hand Contacts

Physical therapists emphasize the importance of precise hand contacts in using PNF. Neurologically, the client wants to push or pull against the contact.

When you place your hands on the **medial** side of the limb, you should be verbally directing the stretcher to push or pull in that direction. Asking for a **lateral** push while holding on the medial side may be very confusing to the stretcher because your verbal commands don't match the proprioceptive cues your hands are communicating.

PART

11

The Stretches

In part I, we looked at the historical development of PNF techniques, their neurophysiological foundation, and the development of techniques like facilitated stretching for use with healthy people. We also looked at the various types of stretching and the importance of using good biomechanics when stretching.

In part II, we teach you, step-by-step, how to stretch each major muscle in the body, both singly and in groups. Chapter 4 covers the hips and legs, chapter 5 is devoted to the shoulder and arm, and chapter 6 details stretches for the neck and torso. Chapter 7 looks at how PNF techniques can be incorporated into a rehabilitation program to restore pain-free motion, flexibility, strength, endurance, and speed.

Spiral Patterns or Single Muscle Stretches

PNF techniques were developed as patterns of spiral movement to increase strength, coordination, and flexibility through entire ranges of motion. Facilitated stretching is based on these principles but focuses on increased flexibility and coordination, not necessarily on the development of strength.

When should you use patterns, and when should you use single muscle stretches? We use the spiral-diagonal patterns as a way to increase the flexibility and coordination of groups of muscles that act together. Using these three-dimensional patterns, we stretch groups of muscles simultaneously, thereby gaining greater benefit in a shorter amount of time compared with the single muscle stretches.

We can also use the patterns as an evaluative tool to determine which muscles in a synergistic group are limiting motion, exhibiting weakness, or not firing in the proper sequence. Once these deficiencies are identified, we can modify the patterns to focus on improving the muscular function that needs work.

We use single muscle, or single plane, stretches when we want to develop flexibility or awareness in a specific muscle or muscle group. Single muscle stretches can also be used as an adjunct to soft tissue therapy. For instance, you can use these stretches for relaxing hypertonic (too tight) muscles to reduce the discomfort of deep massage or trigger-point work or in conjunction with deep friction work to release adhesions within or between muscles. (See Appendix A for more on this.)

Organization of Stretches

We've divided each chapter into single muscle stretches and spiral-diagonal patterns, although you may find yourself mixing patterns and single stretches when the need arises. The format for the stretches provides you with the information you need to do them effectively and safely.

Each muscle group is presented as follows:

- Origin, insertion, and action of the muscle(s), with illustrations
- Functional assessment for normal range of motion
- Detailed stretching instructions, with illustrations
- Self-stretching instructions, where appropriate, with illustrations

Some exercise descriptions require special safety notes. Those are indicated with a special symbol. The symbols you see throughout the exercises in part II are explained here. Please adhere to these special notes and cautions when doing any stretch.

Stop movement.   An isometric contraction is one in which no movement occurs. The stretcher begins slowly and builds the contraction as you provide matching resistance, only to your level of strength. Don't allow the stretcher to overpower you. In some cases, the stretcher may be using only 10% of his strength, in other cases, 100%. It all depends on how strong you are in relation to the stretcher. Once the stretcher has achieved the proper level of isometric contraction, hold it for 6 to 10 seconds.

Don't push or pull.   The partner should *never push or pull* to deepen the stretch.

Stretch pain free.   Facilitated stretches should *always be pain free*. If the stretcher experiences pain, try repositioning the limb or use less force during the isometric contraction of the target muscle. If pain persists, don't use facilitated stretching for that particular muscle until you've determined why it's causing pain.

Special notes and cautions.

Chapter 4

Stretches for the Lower Extremity

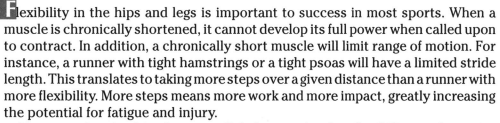

Flexibility in the hips and legs is important to success in most sports. When a muscle is chronically shortened, it cannot develop its full power when called upon to contract. In addition, a chronically short muscle will limit range of motion. For instance, a runner with tight hamstrings or a tight psoas will have a limited stride length. This translates to taking more steps over a given distance than a runner with more flexibility. More steps means more work and more impact, greatly increasing the potential for fatigue and injury.

The stretches in this chapter will help you develop flexibility in the major muscles of the hips and legs, which will contribute to improved athletic performance and more comfort in your daily activities.

HAMSTRINGS
Anatomy

Chronically shortened hamstrings can contribute to low back pain, knee pain, and leg length differences. They can also restrict stride length in walking or running, which means that more work is required to cover a given distance. Runners often have short, weak hamstrings.

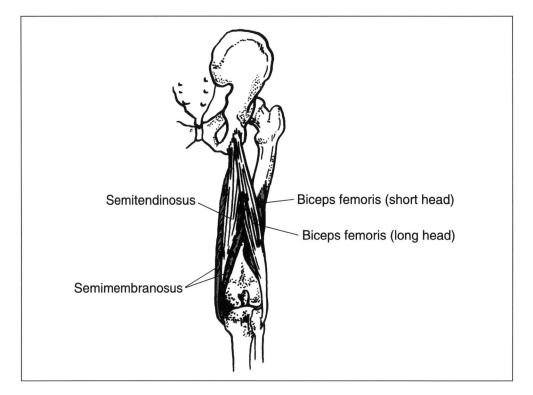

		Origin	Insertion	Action
Hamstrings	Biceps femoris	Long head: ischial tuberosity Short head: linea aspera of femur	Head of the fibula	Long head: hip extension Both heads: knee flexion, lateral rotation of lower leg with knee flexed
	Semimembranosus, Semitendinosus	Ischial tuberosity	Semimembranosus: posteromedial tibial condyle Semitendinosus: anterior proximal tibial shaft (pres anserine)	Hip extension Knee flexion Medial rotation of lower leg with knee flexed

Functional Assessment

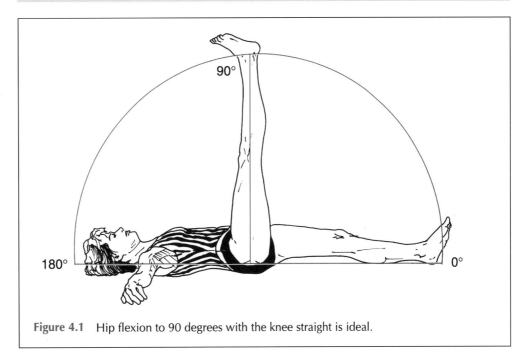

Figure 4.1   Hip flexion to 90 degrees with the knee straight is ideal.

Check range of motion (figure 4.1). Hip flexion to 90 degrees with the leg straight is optimal.

If range is less than 90 degrees, do facilitated stretching for the hamstrings.

Straight Leg Hamstrings Stretch

This is an effective, general stretch for the hamstrings that increases hip flexion.

1. The stretcher is **supine.** He lifts his right leg, with his knee straight, as high as possible. He must keep both hips flat on the table. This lengthens the right hamstrings to their pain-free end of range. As the partner, your job is to gently hold the knee straight as the stretcher lifts.

2. Position yourself to offer resistance to the isometric contraction of the hamstrings (figure 4.2). The stretcher must keep his hips flat on the table during the entire sequence. You may need to work with the stretcher on body awareness, until he is able to stabilize his hips properly, before performing this stretch. The stretcher may bend his left knee and rest his foot flat on the table, instead of having his left leg outstretched if this is a more comfortable position.

3. Direct the stretcher to begin slowly to attempt to push his heel toward the table, isometrically contracting the hamstrings. ("Push against me as if you're trying to put your heel on the table.")

4. After the isometric push, the stretcher relaxes and inhales deeply. During this time, maintain the leg in the starting position.

5. On the exhale, the stretcher contracts the hip flexors (quads and psoas) to lift the leg higher, keeping his knee straight. This deepens the hamstrings stretch. As the stretcher lifts his leg higher, gently hold the knee straight.

6. Now move into the new position to once again offer resistance.

7. Repeat 2 to 3 times.

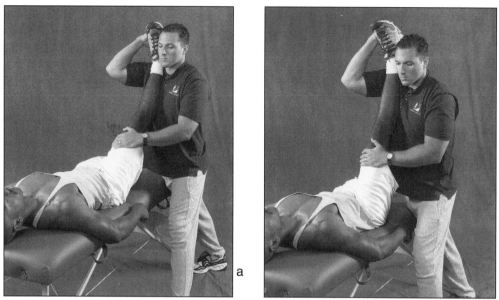

Figure 4.2 (a) Starting position of the straight leg hamstrings stretch (right leg). (b) The stretcher actively deepens the stretch while the partner holds the knee straight.

Bent Knee Hamstrings Stretch

This is a better stretch for people with very short hamstrings. Once they've achieved more flexibility, you can use the straight leg stretch.

1. The stretcher lies supine and lifts his thigh to flex his hip to 90 degrees, with the knee bent.

2. Stabilize the thigh in this position while the stretcher straightens the lower leg as far as possible, without pain. This lengthens the hamstrings to their pain-free end of range (figure 4.3).

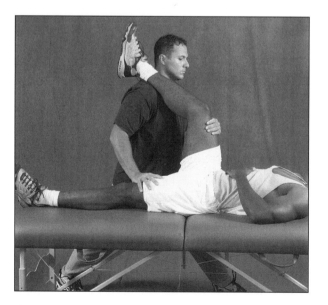

Figure 4.3 Bent knee hamstrings stretch, starting position (right leg).

3. Position yourself to offer resistance to the isometric contraction of the hamstrings, at the same time making sure that the stretcher keeps his hips on the table. The stretcher must keep his hips flat on the table during the entire sequence. You may need to work with the stretcher on body awareness until he is able to stabilize his hips properly before performing this stretch.

4. Direct the stretcher to begin slowly to attempt to push his heel toward the table, bending the knee, which isometrically contracts the hamstrings. ("Keep your thigh where it is, and try to bend your knee by pushing your heel toward the table.")

5. After the isometric push, the stretcher relaxes and inhales deeply. During this time, maintain the leg in the starting position.

6. On the exhale, the stretcher contracts his quadriceps to straighten the leg farther. This deepens the hamstrings stretch. As the stretcher straightens his leg, gently hold the thigh in the 90-degree position.

7. Repeat 2 to 3 times.

Hamstrings Self-Stretch

For self-stretching, the sequence of steps is the same as for assisted stretching, but the partner is replaced by a towel, a strap, or an upright object such as a doorjamb.

- Use a towel wrapped around your heel to provide resistance to the hamstrings contraction. The towel simply replaces the partner. Never pull on the towel to deepen the stretch (figure 4.4).

- Figure 4.5 illustrates another option for self-stretching. Lie in a doorway and use the doorjamb to provide resistance to the hamstrings contraction, then move forward following each round of stretching.

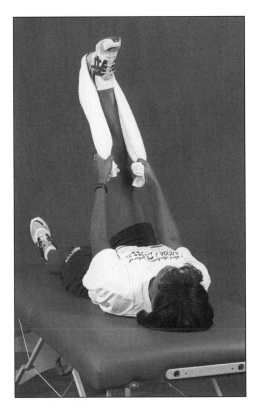

Figure 4.4   Hamstrings self-stretch with a towel.

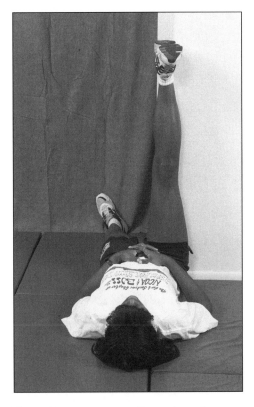

Figure 4.5   Hamstrings self-stretch in a doorway.

QUADRICEPS GROUP
Anatomy

The quadriceps consist of four muscles and are powerful extensors of the knee. One of the quads, the rectus femoris, also crosses the hip joint and acts as a hip flexor, assisting the psoas. Chronically short quads can contribute to low back pain. The quads are usually involved in any type of knee pain or instability.

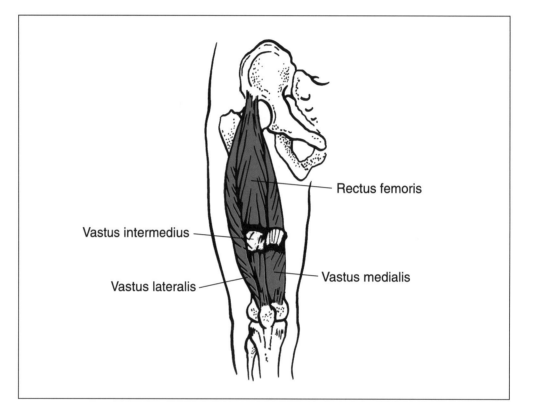

		Origin	Insertion	Action
Quadriceps	Rectus femoris	Anterior inferior iliac spine and upper margin of acetabulum	Patella and via the patellar ligament to tibial tuberosity	Knee extension, assists hip flexion
	Vastus medialis, lateralis, and intermedius	Medialis and lateralis: linea aspera of posterior femur Intermedius: anterior and lateral shaft of femur	Patella and via the patellar ligament to tibial tuberosity	Knee extension

Functional Assessment

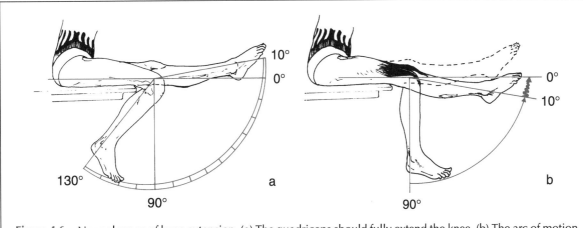

Figure 4.6   Normal range of knee extension. (a) The quadriceps should fully extend the knee. (b) The arc of motion should be smooth, with no hesitation or jerking.

Check range of motion. The quadriceps extend (straighten) the knee.

The stretcher is seated, with legs dangling over the edge of the table. As the stretcher straightens the lower leg, the arc of motion should be smooth and the knee should extend to 0 degrees or beyond into a few degrees of **hyperextension** (figure 4.6).

While on her stomach, the stretcher should be able to bring the heel to the buttock, with a little help from you (figure 4.7). If range is limited, it may be due to tight quads,

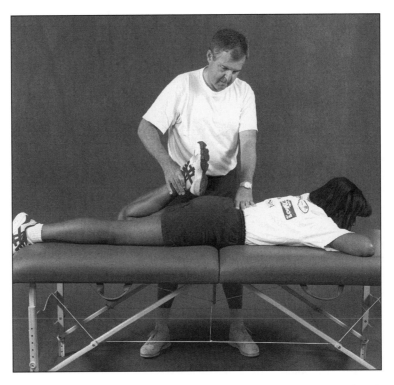

Figure 4.7   The stretcher should be able to bring her heel to her buttock with a little help.

which will be somewhat uncomfortable as you press the heel toward the buttock, or limitation may be due to the bulk of the hamstrings and calf muscles. Facilitated stretching works quite well here if the limitation is due to tight quads.

Quadriceps Stretch

This stretch is used to improve knee flexion.

1. The stretcher lies **prone,** with the knee flexed as far as possible. Because of the bulk of the hamstrings and calf muscles, you may gently push against the leg to bring the heel closer to the buttocks. Push only until the stretcher feels the quads beginning to stretch. This is the pain-free end of range.

If this position causes any low back discomfort, stop and place a pillow under the stretcher's hips to reduce the stress on the low back and begin again. Or, you may want to have the stretcher contract his abdominal muscles to stabilize and flatten his low back. This position can also eliminate low back discomfort.

2. Position yourself to offer resistance to the isometric contraction of the quads by placing your hands or shoulder against the stretcher's shin (figure 4.8). The stretcher must keep his hips flat on the table (or on the pillow) during the entire sequence. You may need to work with the stretcher on body awareness until he is able to stabilize his hips properly before performing this stretch.

3. Direct the stretcher to begin slowly to try to straighten his leg, isometrically contracting the quads.

4. After the isometric push, the stretcher relaxes and inhales deeply. During this time, maintain the leg in the starting position.

5. On the exhale, the stretcher contracts the hamstrings, and you may once again offer assistance by pushing on the leg, deepening the quad stretch.

Occasionally, the hamstrings will go into spasm at this point, possibly because they are contracting from a new, shortened position. Stretching the hamstrings prior to the

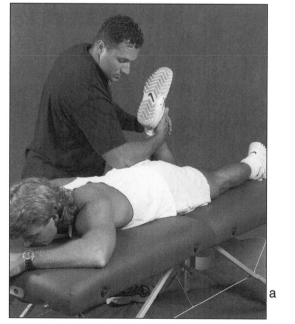 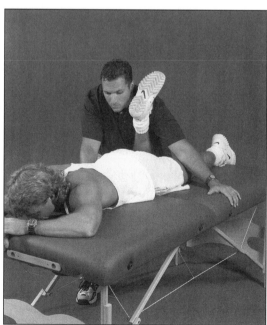

Figure 4.8 Offering resistance to the isometric contraction of the quadriceps. (a) Support the stretcher's leg with your hands. (b) Support the stretcher's leg with your shoulder.

quads usually prevents this problem. As a further precaution, you may instruct the stretcher to only briefly contract the hamstrings (step 5) and then release them while you stretch the quads passively.

6. Repeat 2 to 3 times.

Quadriceps Self-Stretch

Assume the same beginning position as in step 1 of the quadriceps stretch. Use your opposite hand to hold the leg and provide resistance (right hand to left leg, or left hand to right leg). This prevents excessive stress on the medial collateral ligament (figure 4.9a). You may also use a towel wrapped around your leg if this is easier (figure 4.9b).

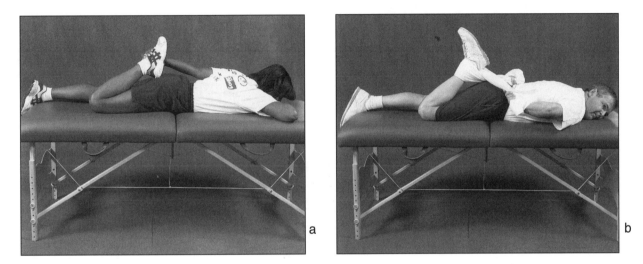

a   b

Figure 4.9 Quadriceps self-stretch. (a) The stretcher holds her leg with her opposite arm. (b) Self-stretch using a towel.

PSOAS AND ILIACUS
Anatomy

The iliopsoas is the primary hip flexor. Because of its attachment along the lumbar spine, it affects the angle of the lumbar curve. If the psoas is too tight, it can cause an increase in the curve, which leads to swayback and low back pain. Conversely, sometimes a tight psoas will flatten the lumbar curve, which can also lead to low back pain. For a more detailed discussion of this seeming contradiction, see Tom Myers' article "Poise: Psoas-Piriformis Balance" (1998).

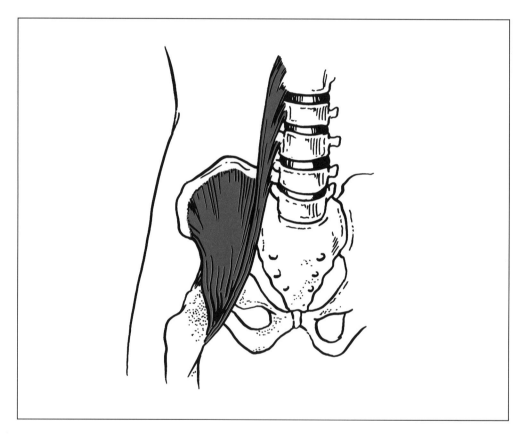

		Origin	Insertion	Action
Iliopsoas	Iliopsoas	Psoas: anterior lumbar vertebrae Iliacus: inner surface of ilium	Lesser trochanter of femur	Flexion and lateral rotation of the femur. Experts disagree on whether it acts as an abductor or adductor.

Functional Assessment

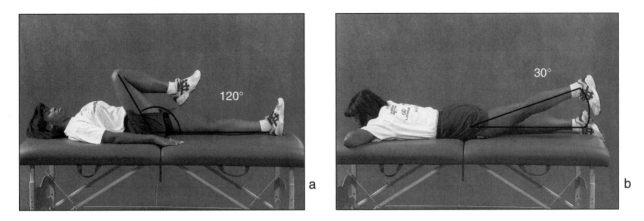

Figure 4.10   Normal range of hip (a) flexion and (b) extension.

Check hip range of motion. Normal range of flexion (120 degrees) allows the stretcher to bring her flexed knee to her chest (figure 4.10a). Normal range in extension is approximately 30 degrees (figure 4.10b).

Modified Thomas Test

To check for tightness in the psoas and/or quadriceps, the stretcher lies supine with the lower legs dangling off the edge of the table, then lifts the right leg, knee to chest.

Check to see whether the stretcher's left lower leg straightens. This indicates tight quadriceps (especially rectus femoris) and tensor fascia latae (TFL) on the left leg (figure 4.11a). If the stretcher's left thigh lifts off the table (figure 4.11b), this indicates a tight iliopsoas on the left.

Repeat for the other leg. It's common for both the quads and the iliopsoas to be hypertonic on the same leg. If the quads are too tight, do facilitated stretching for the quads. If the iliopsoas is too tight, do facilitated stretching for the iliopsoas.

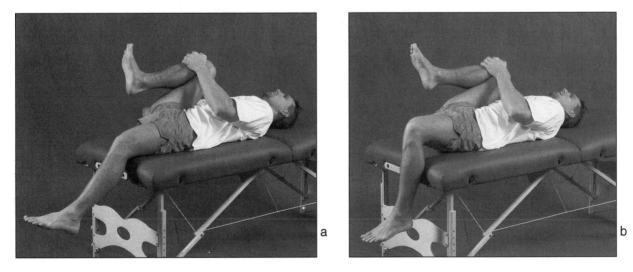

Figure 4.11   Modified Thomas test for psoas and quadriceps tightness. (a) The stretcher flexes his right hip and knee, bringing the knee to the chest. The left lower leg extends, indicating a tight quadriceps, and possibly a tight tensor fascia latae, on the left. (b) The left thigh lifts off the table, indicating a tight psoas on the left.

Iliopsoas Stretch—Prone

This stretch is used to improve hip extension.

1. The stretcher lies prone. If the stretcher has any low back discomfort in this position, place a pillow under his hips to take some of the stress off the low back. Or you may want the stretcher to contract his abdominal muscles to stabilize and flatten his low back. This position can also eliminate low back discomfort.

2. The stretcher uses his hip extensors (gluteals and hamstrings) to lift his leg off the table as high as possible, with the knee bent. This lengthens the iliopsoas to its end of range. The stretcher must keep his hips flat on the table (or on the pillow) throughout this stretch. There will be a strong tendency for him to lift his hip as he lifts his leg. You may need to work with the stretcher on body awareness until he is able to stabilize his hips properly before performing this stretch.

3. Support the leg just above the knee to provide resistance to the isometric contraction of the iliopsoas. Use your hand or your leg to support the stretcher (figure 4.12).

4. Direct the stretcher to begin slowly to try to pull his thigh toward the table, isometrically contracting the iliopsoas. He is not trying to straighten his lower leg.

5. After the isometric push, the stretcher relaxes and inhales deeply. During this time, maintain the leg in the starting position.

6. On the exhale, the stretcher contracts the hip extensors to lift his thigh higher, deepening the psoas stretch. Be sure the stretcher keeps his hips flat on the table.

7. Repeat 2 to 3 times.

8. If you use your leg to provide resistance, move it closer to the hip with each round of stretching (figure 4.13).

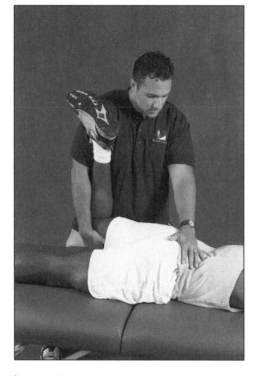

Figure 4.12   Initiation of the prone iliopsoas stretch.

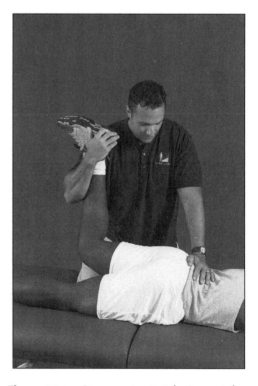

Figure 4.13   Prone psoas stretch. Support the stretcher's leg with your thigh.

Iliopsoas Stretch—Supine

This stretch is used to improve hip extension.

1. The stretcher lies supine with both hips flexed and the greater trochanter of the femur at the end of the table. This position prevents limitation of hip extension by the table.

2. The stretcher holds his right knee to his chest to keep the low back flat on the table. (This is very important for protecting the low back, especially in people with a history of low back pain.) The stretcher may use his hands to hold his right leg up, or he may rest his right foot against you. The stretcher presses his left heel toward the floor, using the hip extensors (gluteals and hamstrings). This lengthens the left iliopsoas to its end of range (figure 4.14).

3. Position yourself to offer resistance to the isometric contraction of the left iliopsoas by applying pressure with your right hand just above the stretcher's left knee. The stretcher must keep his low back flat on the table.

4. Direct the stretcher to begin slowly to try to pull his left leg toward his left shoulder, isometrically contracting the psoas. ("Try to bring your knee toward the ceiling; don't try to straighten your lower leg.")

5. After the isometric push, the stretcher relaxes and inhales deeply. As he relaxes, the left leg may drop of its own accord. On the exhale, the stretcher contracts the hip extensors (gluteals and hams) to press his left heel toward the floor, deepening the iliopsoas stretch. Never push to deepen the stretch.

6. Repeat 2 to 3 times.

7. The stretcher may attempt to recruit his adductors by externally rotating his left leg (figure 4.15). Do not allow this.

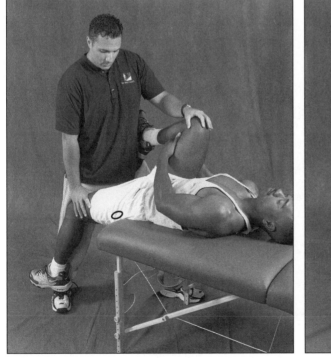

Figure 4.14 Supine iliopsoas stretch, initiation. The greater trochanter is at the edge of the table. Resist the stretcher's effort with your right hand.

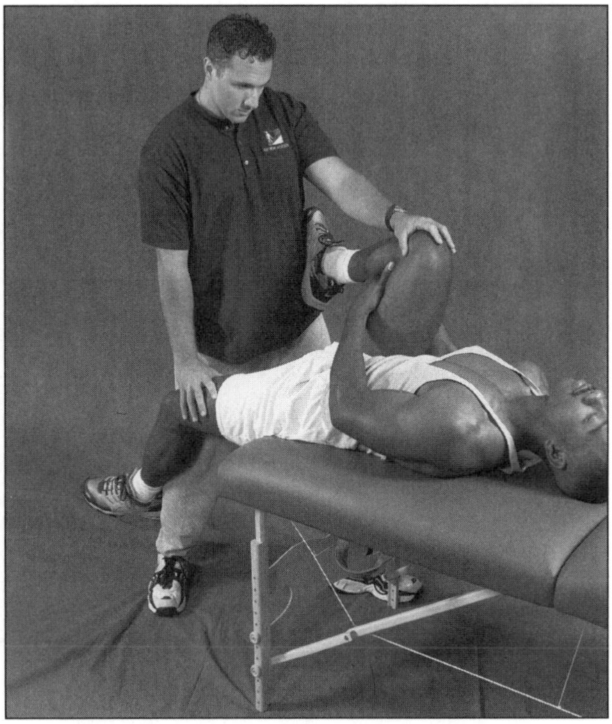

Figure 4.15 The stretcher's left leg is incorrectly externally rotated in an attempt to recruit the adductors.

8. To avoid having the stretcher arch his low back (and to prevent possible low back pain), when you finish stretching the left side, help the stretcher bring both knees to his chest, then lower the right leg to stretch the right iliopsoas. When both sides are finished, help the stretcher bring both knees to his chest. The stretcher then pushes himself more fully onto the table by pushing against you with both feet, then sits up carefully (figure 4.16).

Iliopsoas Self-Stretch

A widely used standing stretch can easily be modified to become a facilitated stretch for the iliopsoas.

1. Stand with your left leg forward and right leg back, keeping your torso upright and your low back flat.

2. Keeping your right foot flat on the floor, push forward with your right hip to lengthen the right iliopsoas. Allow your left knee to bend as you push forward. You should feel the stretch high on the front of the right thigh (figure 4.17).

3. Isometrically contract the right iliopsoas by attempting to pull your right leg forward but keeping the foot anchored on the floor. Be sure your gluteal muscles are relaxed! Maintain the isometric contraction for 6 to 10 seconds, then relax.

4. You can now stretch the iliopsoas by pushing the right hip forward again, being sure to maintain an upright posture with your low back flat.

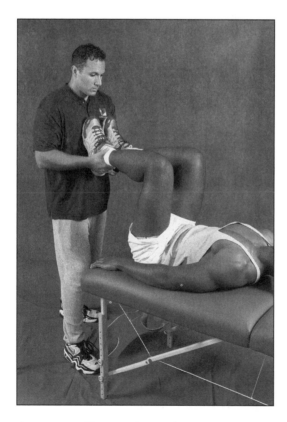

Figure 4.16 The stretcher pushes against you to slide farther onto the table before sitting up.

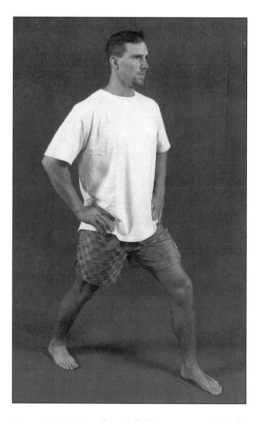

Figure 4.17 Standing right iliopsoas self-stretch. Keep your low back flat and focus on feeling a stretch at the front of your right thigh.

TIBIALIS ANTERIOR
Anatomy

When the foot is free to move, tibialis anterior dorsiflexes and inverts it. When the foot is on the ground, tibialis anterior assists in maintaining balance. During walking or running, it helps prevent the foot from slapping onto the ground after heel-strike and lifts the foot to clear the ground as the leg is swinging forward.

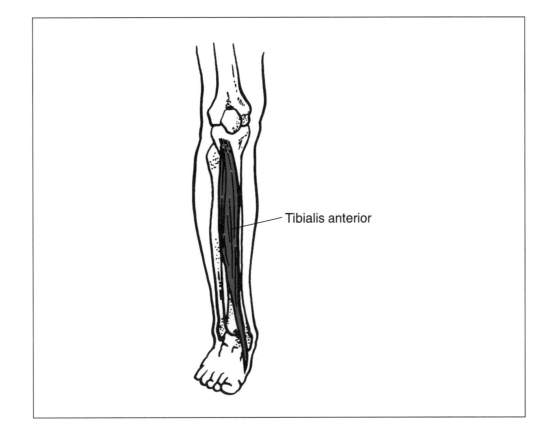

Tibialis anterior

		Origin	Insertion	Action
Tibialis Anterior	Tibialis anterior	Lateral shaft of tibia, interosseous membrane	Base of first metatarsal, first cuneiform	Ankle dorsiflexion Inversion of foot Supports longitudinal arch

Functional Assessment

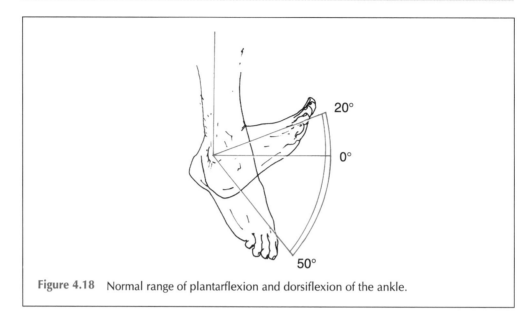

Figure 4.18 Normal range of plantarflexion and dorsiflexion of the ankle.

Check range of motion (figure 4.18). Plantarflexion of the ankle should be approximately 50 degrees. Dorsiflexion of the ankle should be approximately 20 degrees. If range of motion is limited, PNF stretching may be helpful.

Tibialis Anterior Stretch

This stretch is used to improve plantarflexion.

1. The stretcher lies supine and plantarflexes his right ankle (points toes) using the calf muscles. This lengthens the right tibialis anterior to its end of range.

2. Cup the right heel with your left hand and hold the top of the right foot with your right hand (figure 4.19). When stretching the left side, cup the left heel with your right hand and hold the top of the left foot with your left hand.

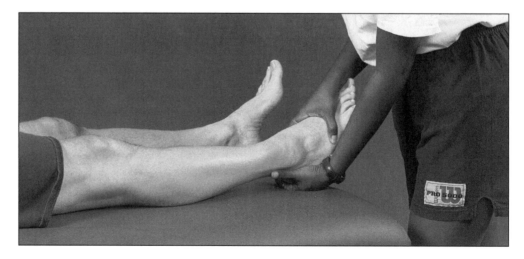

Figure 4.19 Initiation of the tibialis anterior stretch (right foot).

3. Direct the stretcher to begin slowly to attempt to pull his foot toward his knee (dorsiflexion), isometrically contracting the tibialis anterior.

4. After the isometric pull, the stretcher relaxes and inhales deeply. During this time, maintain the foot in the starting position.

5. On the exhale, the stretcher contracts the calf muscles to increase plantarflexion, deepening the tibialis anterior stretch.

6. Repeat 2 to 3 times.

Tibialis Anterior Self-Stretch

For self-stretching, the sequence of steps is the same as for the assisted stretch. Your foot can be plantarflexed and then anchored under a couch, a bed, or the strap of a sit-up bench to provide resistance to the isometric contraction. You can also sit on your heels and use the floor to resist the isometric contraction (figure 4.20).

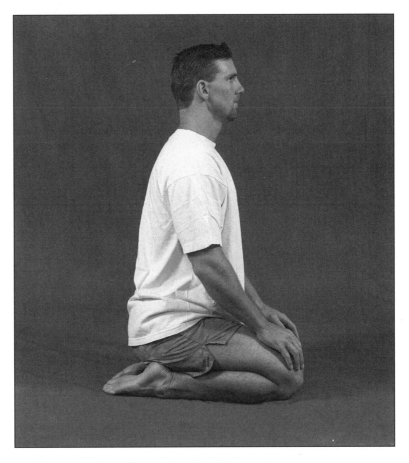

Figure 4.20   Sitting self-stretch for the tibialis anterior.

GASTROCNEMIUS-SOLEUS
Anatomy

The gastrocnemius-soleus muscles are also called the "triceps surae." They insert into the heel via the Achilles tendon, the strongest tendon in the body. The gastrocnemius is a two-headed muscle that gives the calf its shape. The soleus muscle, which lies underneath the gastrocnemius, is more often the reason for calf tightness.

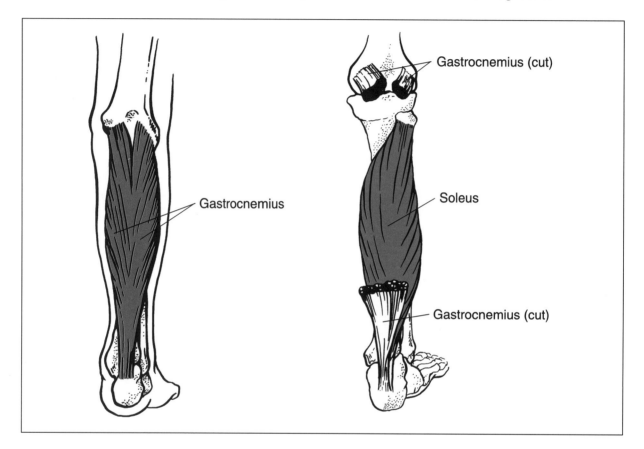

		Origin	Insertion	Action
Gastrocnemius	Gastrocnemius	Medial head: medial epicondyle of femur Lateral head: lateral epicondyle of femur	Calcaneus via the Achilles tendon	Plantarflexion of ankle or assists flexion of knee, but cannot do both simultaneously
Soleus	Soleus	Soleal line of tibia and posterior head and upper shaft of fibula	Calcaneus via the Achilles tendon	Plantarflexion of ankle (stronger plantarflexion than gastrocnemius)

Functional Assessment

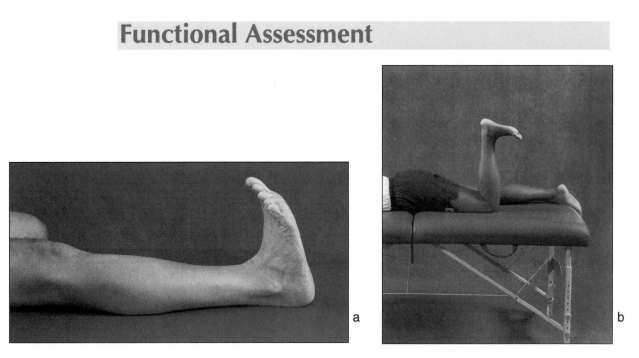

Figure 4.21   (a) Normal range of dorsiflexion of the ankle. (b) With the knee bent, the gastrocnemius is slack and any limitation in dorsiflexion is due to a tight soleus.

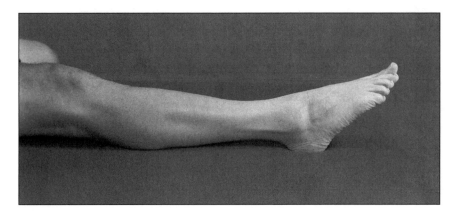

Figure 4.22   Normal range of plantarflexion of the ankle.

Check range of motion. Dorsiflexion should be approximately 20 degrees (figure 4.21a).

If dorsiflexion is limited, have the stretcher lie prone and flex the knee to 90 degrees and test again (figure 4.21b). Knee flexion relaxes the gastrocnemius and eliminates it as a limiter of dorsiflexion. So if limitation is still present after flexing the knee, focus the stretching on the soleus. If knee flexion improves dorsiflexion, focus the stretching on the gastrocnemius.

Plantarflexion should be 50 degrees (figure 4.22). Limited plantarflexion may be due to a tight tibialis anterior.

Gastrocnemius-Soleus Stretch—Supine

This stretch is used to improve dorsiflexion.

1. The stretcher lies supine, legs straight, and lightly grips the sides of the table to keep from sliding during the isometric phase.

GASTROCNEMIUS-SOLEUS

2. The stretcher dorsiflexes his right foot (brings the foot toward the knee) as far as possible (figure 4.23). This lengthens the gastroc/soleus to its end of range.

● 3. Stand at the end of the table and place both hands around the stretcher's foot. Use your body weight to offer resistance to the isometric contraction of the gastroc/soleus as you direct the stretcher to begin slowly to attempt to plantarflex (push the foot toward you), isometrically contracting the gastroc-soleus.

4. After the isometric push, the stretcher relaxes and inhales deeply. During this time, maintain the foot in the starting position.

5. On the exhale, the stretcher contracts the tibialis anterior, dorsiflexing the foot and deepening the gastroc-soleus stretch.

6. Repeat 2 to 3 times.

Gastrocnemius-Soleus Stretch—Prone

1. The stretcher lies prone on the table, with his feet hanging over the edge far enough so that he can fully dorsiflex without interference from the table.

2. The stretcher dorsiflexes one foot (brings the foot toward the knee) as far as possible. This lengthens the gastroc-soleus to its end of range.

3. Stand at the end of the table and place the palm of your hand against the stretcher's foot. Use your thigh to support your hand, being sure to maintain good posture (figure 4.24).

Offer resistance as you direct the stretcher to begin slowly to attempt to plantarflex (push the foot toward you), isometrically contracting the gastroc-soleus.

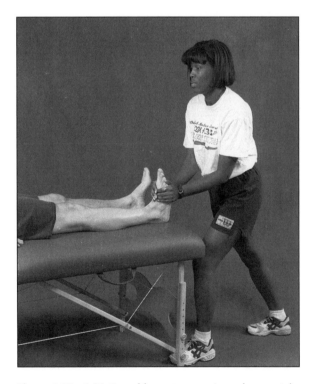

Figure 4.23 Initiation of the gastrocnemius-soleus stretch, supine. Assume a wide stance and resist with both hands.

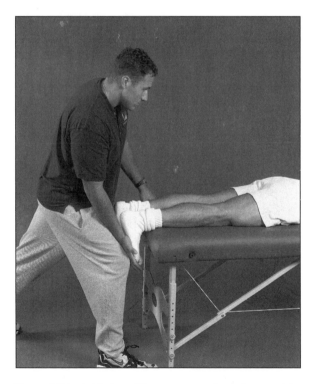

Figure 4.24 Initiation of the gastrocnemius-soleus stretch, prone.

4. After the isometric push, the stretcher relaxes and inhales deeply. During this time, maintain the foot in the starting position.

5. On the exhale, the stretcher contracts the tibialis anterior, dorsiflexing the foot and deepening the gastroc-soleus stretch.

6. Repeat 2 to 3 times.

Soleus Stretch—Prone

This stretch isolates the soleus and is used to improve dorsiflexion.

1. The stretcher lies prone on the table, with one knee flexed to 90 degrees. This position isolates the soleus muscle. He then dorsiflexes his foot (brings the foot toward the knee) as far as possible. This lengthens the soleus to its end of range.

2. Support the bent leg with one hand and wrap your other hand around the heel with your forearm resting against the sole of the foot (figure 4.25a). As another option, sit on the table, interlace your fingers, and place them across the metatarsal arch of the foot (figure 4.25b).

3. Offer resistance as you direct the stretcher to begin slowly to attempt to plantarflex (push the foot toward you), isometrically contracting the soleus.

4. After the isometric push, the stretcher relaxes and inhales deeply. During this time, maintain the foot in the starting position.

5. On the exhale, the stretcher contracts the tibialis anterior, dorsiflexing the foot and deepening the soleus stretch.

6. Repeat 2 to 3 times.

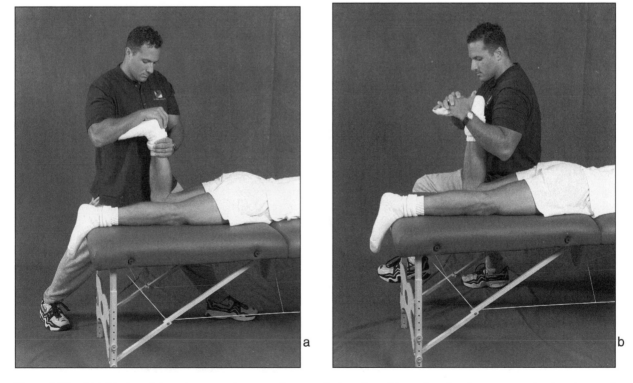

Figure 4.25   (a) Initiation of the soleus stretch, prone. Support the bent leg with one hand and wrap your other hand around the heel, with your forearm resting against the sole of the foot. (b) Or, sit on the table, interlace your fingers, and place them across the metatarsal arch of the foot.

GASTROCNEMIUS-SOLEUS

GASTROCNEMIUS-SOLEUS

Gastrocnemius-Soleus Self-Stretch

Sit with your leg straight, a towel wrapped around your foot and held in both hands to provide resistance during the isometric phase (figure 4.26).

Soleus Self-Stretch

Sit with your knee bent, and use your hands or a towel to provide resistance during the isometric phase (figure 4.27).

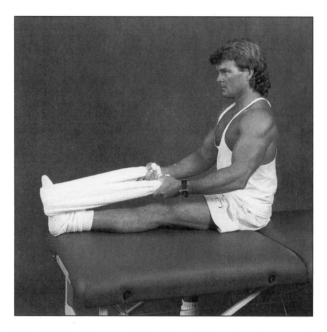

Figure 4.26 Gastrocnemius-soleus self-stretch, using a towel.

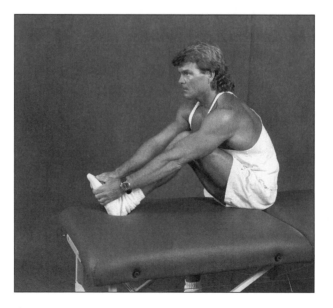

Figure 4.27 Soleus self-stretch, knee bent.

PERONEALS AND TIBIALIS POSTERIOR
Anatomy

Eversion (pronation) and inversion (supination) of the foot occur with every step in walking or running. Proper function of the evertors and invertors of the foot is critical for maintaining good biomechanics of the foot and ankle, as well as for stabilizing the leg on the foot. Like many of the lower limb muscles, the invertors and evertors often act to control movement rather than initiate it.

The primary evertors of the foot are two of the three peroneal muscles: the peroneus longus and the brevis. They make up the lateral compartment of the leg. A third evertor, peroneus tertius, when present at all, is found in the anterior compartment with the tibialis anterior.

Although the peroneals are most often considered to be evertors of the foot, they also function to stabilize the foot, ankle, and leg along with the other muscles of the lower limb.

The primary invertors of the foot are tibialis **anterior** and **posterior**. The tibialis posterior is the deepest muscle in the calf. To review the anatomy and actions of the tibialis anterior, see page 45.

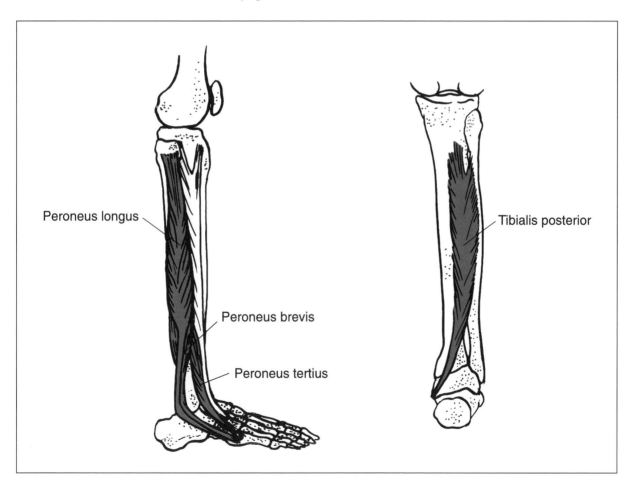

Peroneus longus

Peroneus brevis

Peroneus tertius

Tibialis posterior

PERONEALS AND TIBIALIS POSTERIOR

		Origin	Insertion	Action
Evertors	Peroneus longus	Proximal 2/3 of lateral fibula	Base of first metatarsal and medial cuneiform	Eversion of foot Assists plantarflexion of foot Stabilizes leg on foot Supports medial arch (in conjunction with anterior tibialis)
	Peroneus brevis	Distal 2/3 of lateral fibula (lies deep to peroneus longus)	Peroneal tubercle on lateral aspect of 5th metatarsal	Eversion of foot Assists dorsiflexion
	Peroneus tertius (often absent)	Distal half of anterior fibula	Peroneal tubercle on lateral aspect of 5th metatarsal and base of 4th metatarsal	Eversion of foot Assists dorsiflexion
Invertors	Tibialis anterior	Lateral shaft of tibia, interosseous membrane	Base of first metatarsal, first cuneiform	Ankle dorsiflexion Inversion of foot Supports longitudinal arch
	Tibialis posterior	Interosseous membrane, medial fibula, and posterolateral tibia	Primarily the navicular and medial cuneiform, and also the cuboid, calcaneus, and bases of the second, third, and fourth metatarsals	Inversion of the foot Assists plantarflexion and inversion

Functional Assessment

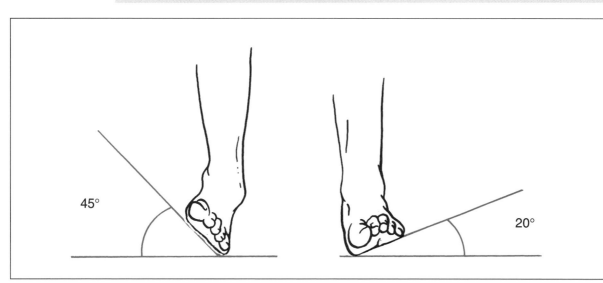

Check range of motion. Eversion (pronation) should be approximately 20 degrees. Inversion (supination) should be approximately 45 degrees.

Evertor (Peroneal) Stretch—Supine

This stretch is used to increase inversion of the ankle.

1. The stretcher lies supine and inverts his right ankle (turns the sole of his foot toward the midline) by contracting the invertors. The ankle is kept in neutral relative to dorsiflexion or plantarflexion. This lengthens the right peroneals to their end of range.

2. Grasp his lower leg with your right hand to stabilize it, and place your left hand against the lateral side (little toe side) of the stretcher's right foot (figure 4.28).

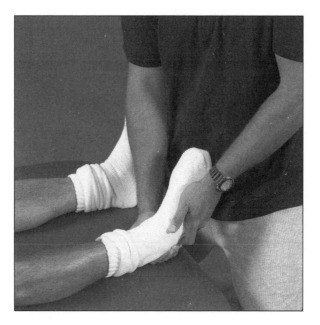

Figure 4.28   Initiation of the peroneal stretch.

PERONEALS AND TIBIALIS POSTERIOR

● 3. Direct the stretcher to begin slowly to attempt to turn the sole of his foot out against your hand (eversion), isometrically contracting the peroneals.

4. After the isometric push, the stretcher relaxes and inhales deeply. During this time, maintain the foot in the starting position.

5. On the exhale, the stretcher contracts the invertors to increase inversion, deepening the peroneal stretch.

6. Repeat 2 to 3 times.

Invertor (Posterior Tibialis) Stretch—Supine

This stretch is used to increase eversion of the ankle.

1. The stretcher lies supine and everts his right ankle (turns the sole of his foot away from the midline) by contracting the peroneal muscles (evertors). The ankle is kept in neutral relative to dorsiflexion or plantarflexion. This lengthens the right posterior tibialis to its end of range.

2. Grasp his lower leg with your left hand to stabilize it, and place your right hand against the medial side (big toe side) of the stretcher's right foot (figure 4.29).

3. Direct the stretcher to begin slowly to attempt to turn the sole of his foot inward against your hand (inversion), isometrically contracting the posterior tibialis.

4. After the isometric push, the stretcher relaxes and inhales deeply. During this time, maintain the foot in the starting position.

5. On the exhale, the stretcher contracts the peroneals to increase eversion, deepening the tibialis posterior stretch.

6. Repeat 2 to 3 times.

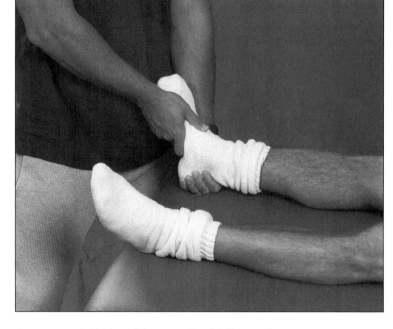

Figure 4.29 Initiation of the posterior tibialis stretch.

HIP ADDUCTORS
Anatomy

The adductor muscles can be divided into short adductors and long adductors. We've provided one illustration showing all the adductors but will treat the two groups separately in the following stretches.

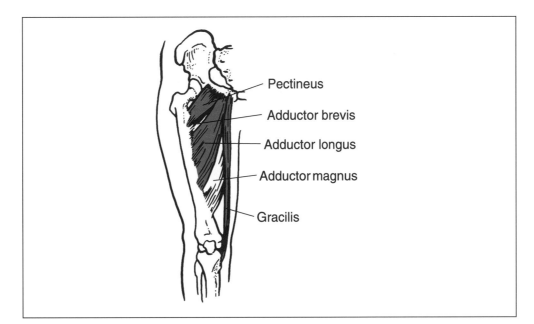

		Origin	Insertion	Action
Short Adductors	Pectineus		Between the lesser trochanter and linea aspera of posterior femur	Hip flexion Assists adduction and lateral rotation of hip
	Adductor brevis and longus	Anterior pubis	Linea aspera of posterior femur	Adduction of hip Assists flexion and lateral rotation of hip
Long Adductors	Adductor magnus	Pubic ramus, ischial tuberosity	Linea aspera of posterior femur Adductor tubercle of medial femur	Powerful adduction of hip The anterior fibers (O on pubic ramus): assist hip flexion The posterior fibers (O on ischial tuberosity): assist hip extension
	Gracilis	Anterior pubis	Medial proximal tibia (pes anserine)	Adduction of hip Assists knee flexion and medial rotation of flexed knee

Functional Assessment

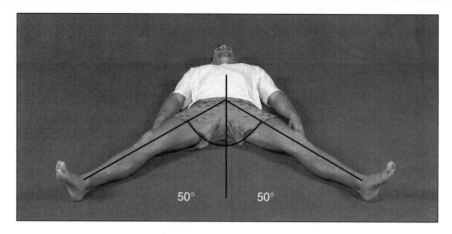

Figure 4.30 Normal range of hip abduction is 45 to 50 degrees from the midline. Limitation is probably due to tight adductors.

Check the range of motion. Normally, the legs should be able to abduct 45 to 50 degrees from the midline (figure 4.30). If this range is limited, it's often due to tight adductors. Use facilitated stretching to increase this range.

▼ The adductors assist hip flexion and help to stabilize the legs in running. They are commonly much tighter in men than in women. Groin pulls are often related to fatigue or improper stretching of the adductor longus.

Supine Stretch for the Short Adductors

This stretch is used to increase abduction.

1. The stretcher is supine on the table. Position yourself to lightly stabilize the stretcher's left hip against the table, using your other hand to control the stretcher's right leg. Direct the stretcher to keep his hips flat on the table during the entire sequence. Your hand is on his left hip as a reminder.

2. The stretcher bends his right knee, places the sole of his right foot against the inside of his left knee, and lowers his right leg toward the table as far as it will go, keeping his left hip flat on the table. This lengthens the short adductors to their end range (figure 4.31).

3. With your hand on the inside of his right knee, direct the stretcher to begin slowly to attempt to push his right knee toward the ceiling, isometrically contracting the short adductors.

4. After the isometric push, the stretcher relaxes and inhales deeply. During this time, maintain the leg in the starting position.

5. On the exhale, the stretcher contracts the hip abductors to pull his knee toward the floor. This deepens the adductor stretch.

6. Repeat 2 to 3 times.

7. After the final stretch, help the stretcher bring his legs together to avoid possible groin strain from this vulnerable position.

8. The stretcher will sometimes get abductor cramps during this stretch. If this occurs, stop and stretch the abductors first, then go back to the adductor stretches.

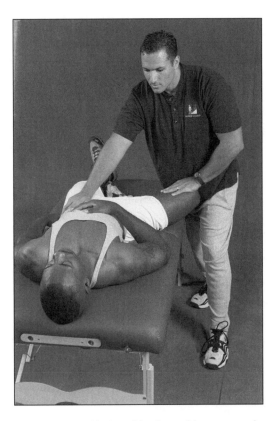

Figure 4.31 Initiation of the short adductors stretch, supine.

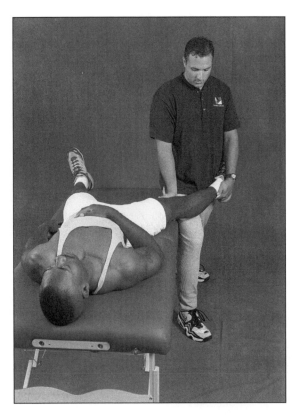

Figure 4.32 Initiation of the long adductors stretch, supine.

Supine Stretch for the Long Adductors

This stretch is used to increase abduction.

1. The stretcher is supine. He abducts his right hip as far as he can, keeping the knee straight and kneecap pointed toward the ceiling (this prevents rotation of the leg). He may hook his left heel over the edge of the table to keep his left leg from sliding across the table. In this position, the long adductors on the right are at the end of their range.

2. Standing at the right side of the table, between the table and the stretcher's leg, support the lower leg with your left hand and place your right hand across the medial aspect of the knee. This position prevents stress to the medial collateral ligament during the isometric phase (figure 4.32).

Ask the stretcher to begin slowly to attempt to bring his right leg toward the midline, isometrically contracting the long adductors.

3. After the isometric push, the stretcher relaxes and inhales deeply. During this time, maintain the leg in the starting position.

4. On the exhale, ask him to abduct his hip farther, deepening the stretch of the long adductors.

5. Repeat 2 to 3 times. After the final stretch, help the stretcher bring his leg back to the table. This helps prevent possible groin strain.

6. Occasionally, the stretcher will experience abductor cramping during this stretch. If this occurs, stop and stretch the abductors, then come back to the adductor stretch.

Short Adductors Self-Stretch

Sit with your back straight, knees bent, and the soles of your feet together. Provide your own resistance to the isometric contraction by using your hands or arms against your medial knees (figure 4.33).

Long Adductors Self-Stretch

This stretch is an adaptation of a common adductors stretch. To stretch the right long adductors, assume a side-lunge position, being careful not to bend the left knee beyond 90 degrees, keeping the right leg straight, foot flat on the floor. All your weight is on your left leg. From this starting position, attempt to pull your right leg toward your midline, using the floor to provide resistance to this movement. After the isometric contraction, deepen the stretch by sinking lower into your left leg (figure 4.34).

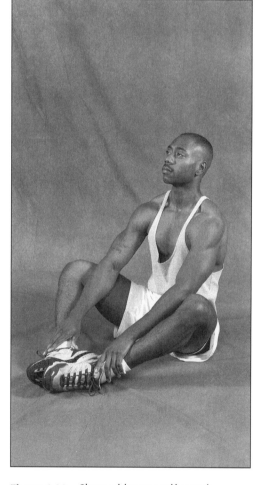

Figure 4.33   Short adductors self-stretch.

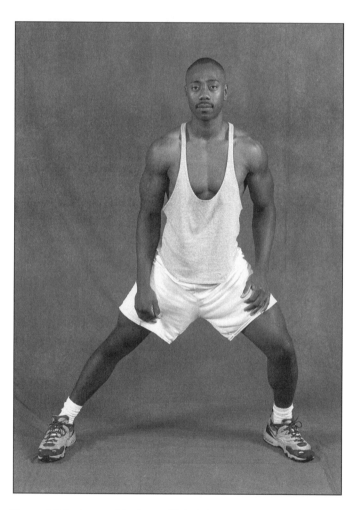

Figure 4.34   Long adductors self-stretch.

HIP ABDUCTORS
Anatomy

The primary abductors of the hip are the tensor fascia latae (TFL) and the gluteus medius and minimus. These muscles not only abduct the hip, they also stabilize it during weight bearing activities. Tightness in these muscles can contribute to pelvic imbalances, which can cause pain not only in the hips, but also in the low back and the knee.

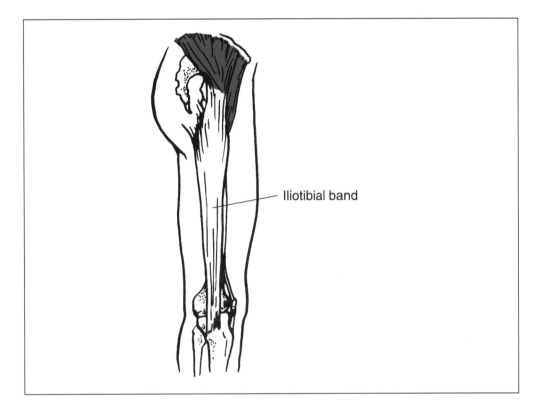

Iliotibial band

		Origin	Insertion	Action
Hip Abductors	Tensor fascia latae (TFL) and iliotibial (IT) band	Iliac crest, just posterior to anterior superior iliac spine	Iliotibial band, which then inserts at lateral tibial condyle (Gerdy's tubercle)	Prevents knee from collapsing during movement Assists abduction, medial rotation and flexion of hip Assists knee extension
	Gluteus medius	Just below crest of ilium, between the anterior and posterior gluteal lines Its posterior 1/3 is covered by gluteus maximus	Posterior superior aspect of greater trochanter	Primary abductor of hip Anterior fibers assist medial rotation and flexion of hip Stabilizes pelvis during walking or running When left leg is in swing phase (non-weight bearing), right gluteus medius contraction prevents pelvis from tilting down on left
	Gluteus minimus	Deep to gluteus medius, attaching along lateral surface of the ilium, between the anterior superior iliac spine and the greater sciatic notch	Anterior superior greater trochanter	Abduction of hip Anterior fibers assist medial rotation and flexion of hip Assists gluteus medius in stabilizing the pelvis

Functional Assessment

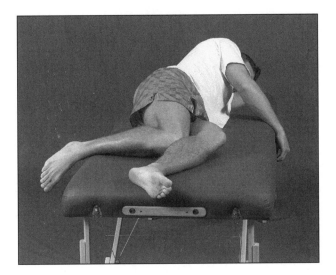

Figure 4.35   Abductor tightness test. Excessive tightness in the hip abductors prevents this position.

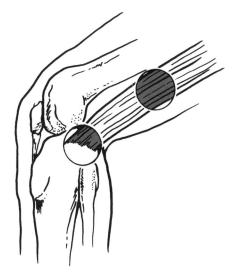

Figure 4.36   IT band syndrome pain sites.

The leg is normally able to swing across the midline of the body about 30 degrees by making slight adjustments in the position of the legs. This motion can be limited by excessive tightness in the hip abductors. Because these muscles also function as knee stabilizers, via the iliotibial (IT) band, knee problems can develop when they are hypertonic (too tight).

To test for this, have the stretcher lie on his side, with the knee of the top leg tucked behind the knee of the other leg (figure 4.35). Excessive tightness in the hip abductors prevents this position and can lead to problems such as IT band syndrome.

▼ IT band syndrome is an overuse injury caused by a tight IT band rubbing over the lateral femoral condyle. It's often found in cyclists and novice runners who overpronate. The pain is normally experienced just proximal to the lateral knee but may also be found at the IT band insertion on the tibia. Figure 4.36 shows the areas of pain. Tightness in the band can be caused by a tight TFL and/or gluteus medius, which pull on the band, or by a hypertrophied vastus lateralis, which bulges under the band and stretches it.

▼ Gluteus medius and minimus are frequently hypertonic and develop trigger points that may cause pain that mimics sciatica or SI joint dysfunction.

Side-Lying Stretch for the Hip Abductors

This stretch is used to improve adduction at the hip.

1. The stretcher is side lying at the edge of the table, top leg hyperextended and hanging over the edge of the table, the bottom leg bent for comfort and stability. The hips are stacked vertically on top of each other. The stretcher contracts his adductors to pull the top leg toward the floor, lengthening the abductors to their end range.

If the stretcher experiences any low back pain in this position, he may bend forward from the waist to round his low back, while keeping his leg hanging off the edge of the table.

2. Stand behind the stretcher to offer support, and stabilize his hip with one hand. With the other hand, offer resistance just above the knee to the isometric contraction of the abductors (figure 4.37).

● 3. Direct the stretcher to begin slowly to try to push his leg toward the ceiling, which isometrically contracts the abductors.

4. After the isometric push, the stretcher relaxes and inhales deeply. As he relaxes, allow the leg to drop toward the floor.

5. On the exhale, the stretcher pulls his leg toward the floor, deepening the abductor stretch even farther.

6. Repeat 2 to 3 times.

Supine Stretch for the Hip Abductors

1. The stretcher is supine, his right leg flat on the table; his left leg is placed over the right, knee bent, and foot flat on the table. He adducts the right leg across the midline as far as possible, keeping the kneecap pointed toward the ceiling to prevent the leg from rolling. This lengthens the right abductors to their end range.

2. Place one hand on the lateral knee of the right leg and stabilize the opposite hip with the other hand to provide resistance to the isometric contraction of the abductors (figure 4.38).

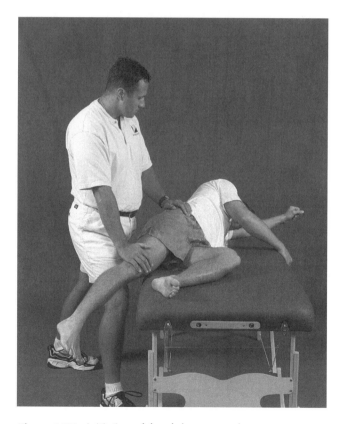

Figure 4.37   Initiation of the abductor stretch.

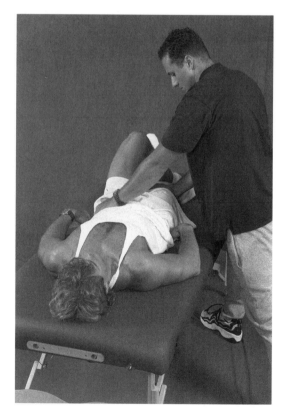

Figure 4.38   Initiation of the abductor stretch, supine.

3. Direct the stretcher to begin slowly to try to push his leg against your hand, isometrically contracting the abductors.

4. After the isometric push, the stretcher relaxes and inhales deeply. As he relaxes, maintain the leg in the starting position.

5. On the exhale, the stretcher pulls his leg farther across the midline, deepening the abductor stretch.

6. Repeat 2 to 3 times.

Hip Abductors Self-Stretch

An easy self-stretch for the hip abductors can be done in the supine position, illustrated in the preceding stretch. Use your bent leg (step 1) to provide resistance to the target leg during the isometric phase (figure 4.39).

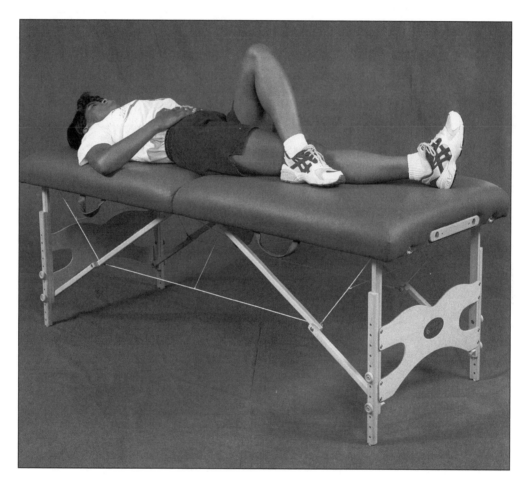

Figure 4.39   Hip abductors self-stretch.

PIRIFORMIS
Anatomy

The piriformis is one of six deep lateral hip rotators, all of which insert on some portion of the greater trochanter. When these muscles are hypertonic, they contribute to a toe-out gait, commonly seen in dancers, and they restrict internal rotation of the hip. Stretching the piriformis also stretches the other lateral rotators.

Note: According to Myers (1998), "Although the piriformis is considered to be a lateral rotator of the hip, its more important function may be as a postural muscle, acting to stabilize the spine, via its attachment on the sacrum, and to maintain pelvic balance in concert with the psoas."

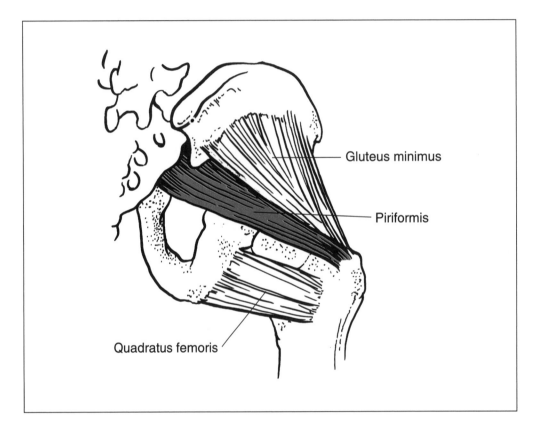

Gluteus minimus

Piriformis

Quadratus femoris

		Origin	Insertion	Action
Piriformis	Piriformis	Anterior sacrum	Superior aspect of greater trochanter	Lateral rotation of femur Assists abduction of femur, especially when hip is flexed May act as medial rotator when hip is hyperflexed Helps stabilize hip joint

Functional Assessment

With client standing relaxed, in bare feet, check for level iliac crests, anterior superior iliac spines (ASIS), and posterior superior iliac spines (PSIS). Also note whether one PSIS is anterior compared with the other. Imbalance in these areas is common with piriformis syndrome.

With the client supine, compare lateral rotation of the legs. Excessive lateral rotation (45 degrees or more) indicates piriformis shortening on that side.

▼ Tightness in the lateral rotators, of which the piriformis is one, is a common cause of sciatic pain. The sciatic nerve exits the sciatic notch of the ilium and travels through these muscles on its way to the posterior thigh (figure 4.40). When the muscles are hypertonic, they can squeeze the nerve, causing irritation and pain. You can differentiate this type of sciatica from true sciatica by determining where the pain begins. If shooting or burning pain begins at the lumbar spine and travels down the leg, then it is likely to be true sciatica. If this type of pain begins in the buttocks, it's probably because of piriformis syndrome and responds well to massage and stretching.

▼ Morton's Foot and/or overpronation can cause excessive medial rotation and adduction of the thigh during running and walking, causing the piriformis to be overworked as it attempts to counteract medial rotation. This may lead to hypertonicity. A leg length difference can also contribute to piriformis syndrome.

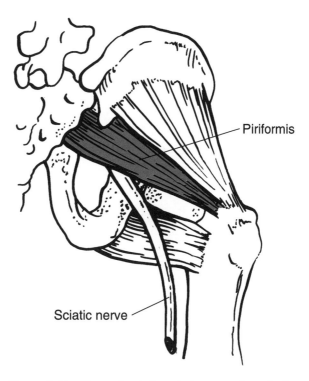

Figure 4.40 The path of the sciatic nerve through the lateral rotators.

PIRIFORMIS

Piriformis Stretch—Supine

This stretch is used to improve medial rotation of the femur. You may have to experiment a little with the starting position of this stretch because each stretcher will feel the muscle stretch in a different position.

1. The stretcher is supine, with right hip and knee flexed to 90 degrees and drawn up toward the left shoulder; the left leg rests on the table. The stretcher then rotates his right thigh laterally by bringing his right foot closer to his left shoulder while maintaining flexion at the hip.

2. Place one hand on the stretcher's lateral knee and the other at his lateral ankle to assist him in finding the leg position that begins to stretch his piriformis. Be sure the stretcher keeps his sacrum on the table. This anchors one end of the piriformis to maximize the stretch. From this starting position, offer resistance to the isometric contraction (figure 4.41).

3. Direct the stretcher to begin slowly to attempt to push his knee and ankle toward you diagonally, isometrically contracting the piriformis.

4. After the isometric push, the stretcher relaxes and inhales deeply. As he relaxes, maintain the leg in the starting position.

5. On the exhale, he contracts his hip flexors and adductors to deepen the piriformis stretch. You may assist by gently pushing to assist hip flexion and adduction, then by adding more lateral rotation to deepen the stretch.

6. Repeat 2 to 3 times.

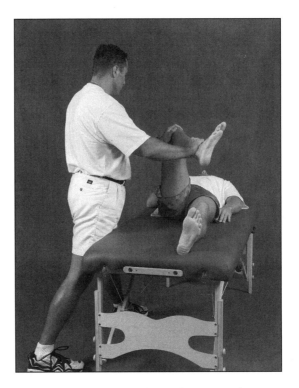

Figure 4.41 Initiation of the piriformis stretch, supine.

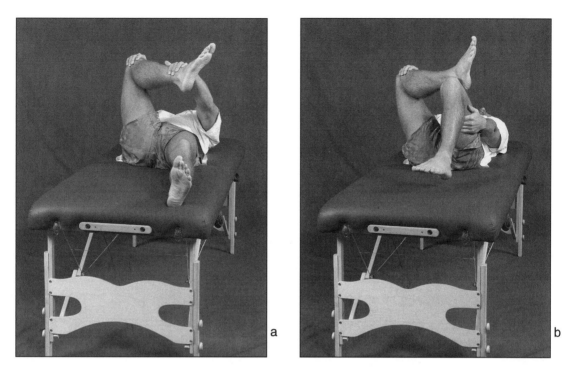

a

b

Figure 4.42 Piriformis self-stretch. (a) Assume the same beginning position as shown in figure 4.41 and use your own hands to provide resistance. (b) Cross the right ankle over the left knee, then bring the left knee toward the left shoulder to begin the stretch of the right piriformis.

Piriformis Self-Stretch

Assume the same beginning position as described in the previous exercise and use your own hands to provide resistance (figure 4.42a).

You may also cross the right ankle over the left knee, then bring the left knee toward the left shoulder being sure to keep the sacrum in contact with the floor or table to begin the stretch of the right piriformis (figure 4.42b).

Spiral Patterns for the Lower Extremity

Not all the spiral patterns for the leg lend themselves to stretching. For instance, the D2 flexion pattern is extremely awkward to carry out. Therefore, we'll be practicing the ones that are the easiest to learn and use. If you have special circumstances with a particular stretcher, feel free to be creative in developing other stretches based on PNF principles and the patterns for the leg.

Because using the patterns requires more concentration from both the stretcher and you, we recommend that you illustrate what you want the stretcher to do by taking him through the pattern passively a few times before attempting to perform the stretch.

Remember that we use only the lengthened range of the pattern. Our goal is to improve range of motion into the lengthened direction, so all isometric effort is done into the shortened range. The stretching occurs as the stretcher moves farther into the lengthened range after the isometric contraction.

You may find it useful to review the leg patterns on pages 25-27 before going on.

D1 Extension (Toe-Off) Stretch

This stretch is for increasing range of motion in flexion, adduction, and external rotation.

1. The stretcher is supine, with his right leg in as much flexion, adduction, and external rotation as possible. His foot is dorsiflexed and inverted, and the toes are extended. This is the starting position for the D1 extension pattern and lengthens the target muscles to their end range. These include hamstrings (especially biceps femoris), gluteals, TFL, gastrocnemius (especially lateral head), soleus, and peroneals.

2. Support and stabilize the leg (figure 4.43). Remember, your hand contacts give the stretcher proprioceptive cues about which way to push or pull. Your hand positions should match your verbal commands.

● 3. Direct the stretcher to begin slowly to try to initiate the D1 extension pattern, beginning with internal rotation, then abduction, then extension. ("Begin by rotating, then kick down and out.") Be sure the stretcher keeps both hips flat on the table.

4. After the isometric push, the stretcher relaxes and inhales deeply. As he relaxes, maintain the leg in the starting position.

5. On the exhale, the stretcher moves the hip farther into flexion, then into adduction, and then into external rotation. Remember, we want a blend of all three directions to keep moving in a diagonal line. He increases dorsiflexion and inversion of the foot and extension of the toes. Support the leg but do not push to deepen the stretch.

▲ 6. Repeat 2 to 3 times.

D2 Extension (Turnout) Stretch

This stretch is used to increase range of motion in flexion, abduction, and internal rotation.

1. The stretcher is supine, with his right leg in as much flexion, abduction, and internal rotation as possible. His foot is dorsiflexed and everted, and the toes are extended. This is the starting position for the D2 extension pattern and lengthens the target muscles to their end range. These include gluteals, hamstrings (especially medial), gastrocnemius (especially medial head), soleus, gracilis, adductors, and posterior tibialis.

2. Support and stabilize the leg (figure 4.44). Remember, your hand contacts give the stretcher proprioceptive cues about which way to push or pull. Your hand positions should match your verbal commands.

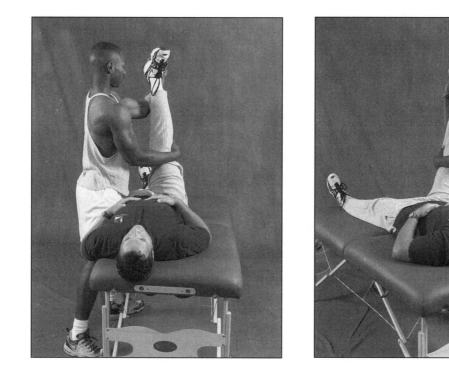

Figure 4.43 Initiation of D1 extension. The right leg is flexed, adducted, and externally rotated.

Figure 4.44 Initiation of D2 extension. The right leg is flexed, abducted, and internally rotated.

3. Direct the stretcher to begin slowly to try to initiate the D2 extension pattern, beginning with external rotation, then adduction, then extension. ("Begin with rotation, then kick down and in.") Be sure the stretcher keeps both hips flat on the table.

4. After the isometric push, the stretcher relaxes and inhales deeply. As he relaxes, maintain the leg in the starting position.

5. On the exhale, the stretcher moves the hip farther into flexion, then into abduction, and then into internal rotation. Remember, we want a blend of all three directions to keep moving in a diagonal line. He increases dorsiflexion and eversion of the foot and extension of the toes.

Support the leg but do not push to deepen the stretch.

6. Repeat 2 to 3 times.

D1 Flexion (Soccer Kick) Stretch

Note: Because the stretcher is prone in this stretch, you may be somewhat confused between internal and external rotation. It may help to pay attention only to the thigh and ignore the position of the lower leg and foot when determining which is internal and which is external rotation.

This stretch is used to improve range of motion into extension, abduction, and internal rotation.

1. The stretcher is prone, with his right knee flexed. Being sure he keeps his hips flat on the table, he lifts his thigh into as much extension, abduction, and internal rotation as possible. For this stretch, the position of the foot and the toes is not important. The knee is in flexion simply to make it easier for the stretcher to lift his leg off the table. If the stretcher experiences any low back discomfort in this position, stop and place a pillow under his hips to make him more comfortable. This is the starting position of D1 flexion

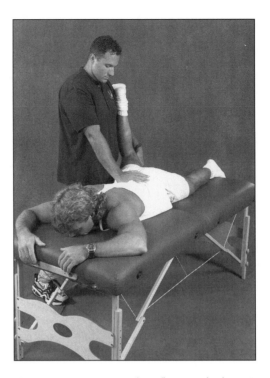

Figure 4.45 Initiation of D1 flexion. The knee is bent, the thigh is extended, abducted, and internally rotated.

and lengthens the target muscles to their end range. These include iliopsoas, rectus femoris, the adductors, and the lateral hip rotators.

2. Support and stabilize the leg, at the same time asking the stretcher to keep both hips on the table (figure 4.45). If the stretcher has enough range of motion, you may be able to support his thigh with your own. If not, use your hand and arm to cradle and support the leg.

3. Direct the stretcher to begin slowly to try to initiate the D1 flexion pattern, beginning with external rotation of the thigh, then adduction, then flexion. ("Begin with rotation, then try to pull down and in.") The stretcher does not try to straighten his knee, only push his thigh toward the table.

4. After the isometric push, the stretcher relaxes and inhales deeply. As he relaxes, maintain the leg in the starting position.

5. On the exhale, the stretcher moves his leg farther into extension, then abduction, and then internal rotation. Remember, we want a blend of all three directions to keep moving in a diagonal line. As he lifts, the stretcher must stabilize his pelvis to keep both hips on the table.

Support the leg but do not assist to deepen the stretch.

6. Repeat 2 to 3 times.

Chapter 5

Stretches for the Upper Extremity

This chapter covers the muscles of the shoulder, arm, and wrist. The shoulder has the greatest range of motion of any joint in the body. We'll look at the four muscles of the rotator cuff, other muscles affecting motion about the shoulder, and the muscles that move the wrist.

ROTATOR CUFF MUSCLES
Anatomy

The tendons of four muscles form the rotator cuff and stabilize the humerus in the glenoid fossa of the scapula during movement.

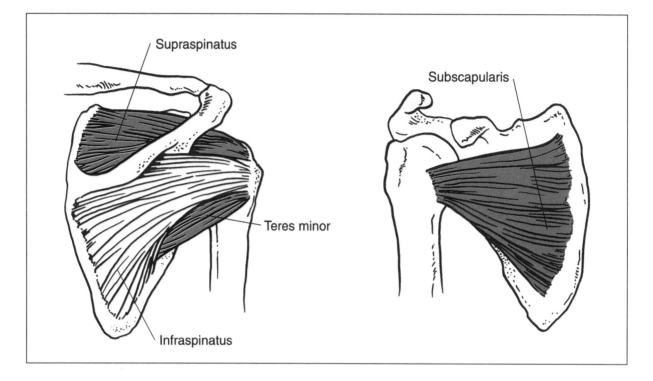

		Origin	Insertion	Action
Rotator Cuff Muscles	Supraspinatus	Supraspinous fossa of scapula	Greater tubercle of humerus (superior facet)	Stabilizes head of humerus in glenoid fossa Initiates abduction
	Infraspinatus	Infraspinous fossa of scapula	Greater tubercle of humerus (middle facet)	Lateral rotation of humerus
	Teres minor	Upper axillary border of scapula	Greater tubercle of humerus (inferior facet)	Lateral rotation of humerus
	Subscapularis	Subscapularis fossa of scapula	Lesser tubercle of humerus	Medial rotation of humerus

Functional Assessment

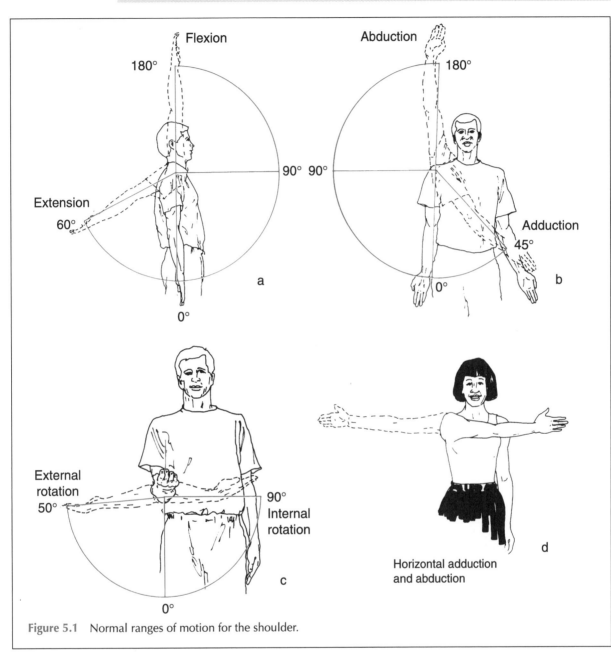

Figure 5.1 Normal ranges of motion for the shoulder.

Active movements can be used to evaluate the entire shoulder complex (humerus, clavicle, scapula) for freedom of movement and for pain. Restriction in range may be limited by hypertrophy or hypertonicity of the muscles or by pain.

Normal ranges of shoulder motion (figure 5.1):

Flexion = 180°	Internal rotation = 90°
Extension = 60°	External rotation = 50°
Adduction = 45°	Horizontal adduction = 130°
Abduction = 180°	Horizontal abduction = 30°

Subscapularis Stretch—Supine

This stretch is used to improve external rotation of the humerus.

1. The stretcher is supine with her shoulder abducted to 90 degrees and her elbow flexed to 90 degrees. Her arm is externally rotated as far as possible and her upper arm is resting completely on the table. This lengthens the subscapularis to its pain-free end of range.

2. Offer resistance to the isometric contraction (no movement) of the subscapularis by placing one hand under the stretcher's elbow and the other hand over her wrist (figure 5.2).

3. Direct the stretcher to begin slowly to attempt to internally rotate her humerus, isometrically contracting the subscapularis. ("Try to push your wrist toward the ceiling.")

4. After the isometric push, the stretcher relaxes and inhales deeply. During this time, maintain the arm in the starting position.

5. On the exhale, the stretcher contracts the infraspinatus to externally rotate the humerus farther, deepening the subscapularis stretch.

6. Repeat 2 to 3 times.

Subscapularis Self-Stretch

An easy stretch for the subscapularis can be done in a doorway. Stand with your arm at your side, the elbow flexed to 90 degrees and the humerus externally rotated as far as possible. It's helpful to think of the arm as a gate that swings back and forth (figure 5.3). Use the doorjamb (or any upright) to resist your attempt to swing the gate closed (the arm pushes toward the stomach).

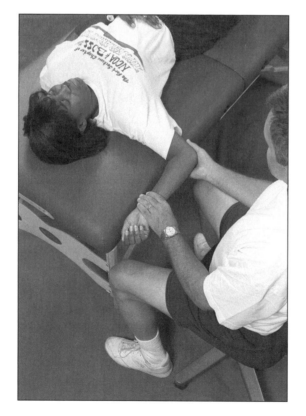

Figure 5.2   Initiation of the subscapularis stretch, supine.

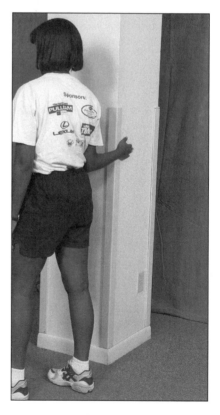

Figure 5.3   Subscapularis self-stretch.

Infraspinatus and Teres Minor Stretch—Prone

This stretch is used to improve internal rotation of the humerus.

1. The stretcher lies prone with his shoulder abducted to 90 degrees and his elbow flexed to 90 degrees. His arm is internally rotated as far as possible and his upper arm is resting completely on the table. (The prone position helps prevent his shoulder from rolling forward, which would give a false impression of the range of internal rotation.) This position lengthens the infraspinatus to its pain-free end of range.

2. Offer resistance to the isometric contraction of the infraspinatus by placing one hand over the stretcher's elbow and the other hand under his wrist (figure 5.4).

3. Direct the stretcher to begin slowly to attempt to externally rotate his humerus, isometrically contracting the infraspinatus. ("Try to push your wrist toward the floor.")

4. After the isometric push, the stretcher relaxes and inhales deeply. During this time, maintain the arm in the starting position.

5. On the exhale, the stretcher contracts the subscapularis to internally rotate the humerus farther, deepening the infraspinatus stretch.

6. Repeat 2 to 3 times.

Infraspinatus and Teres Minor Self-Stretch

The infraspinatus can be a difficult muscle to self-stretch, but here is one option. Assume a "hammerlock" position—that is, with your right arm behind your back and your elbow flexed to approximately 90 degrees. Stand with your back to a door that is closed securely, and grasp the doorknob with your right hand (figure 5.5). Holding the doorknob, try to push your forearm against your back, isometrically contracting the infraspinatus. Following the isometric contraction, pull your forearm farther away from your back as you take a step or two away from the door, still holding onto the doorknob. This stretches the infraspinatus.

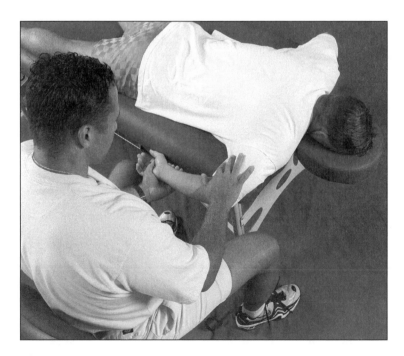

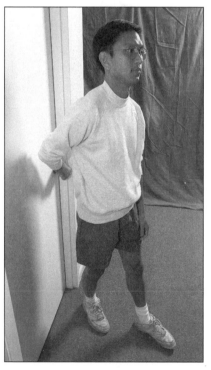

Figure 5.4 Initiation of the infraspinatus stretch, prone. The shoulder and elbow are both at 90 degrees and the upper arm rests on the table.

Figure 5.5 Infraspinatus self-stretch.

PECTORALIS, BICEPS, AND TRICEPS
Anatomy

Three additional muscles affect the shoulder: the biceps brachii, pectoralis major, and triceps. The biceps brachii is a two-headed, two-joint muscle. It crosses both the shoulder and the elbow and affects both. Pectoralis major is a broad, powerful muscle that gives shape to the chest and is a strong mover of the arm. It is divided into two sections: the clavicular head and the sternal head. These two sections have opposite actions. The triceps is a three-headed, two-joint muscle. It crosses both the shoulder and the elbow and acts on both.

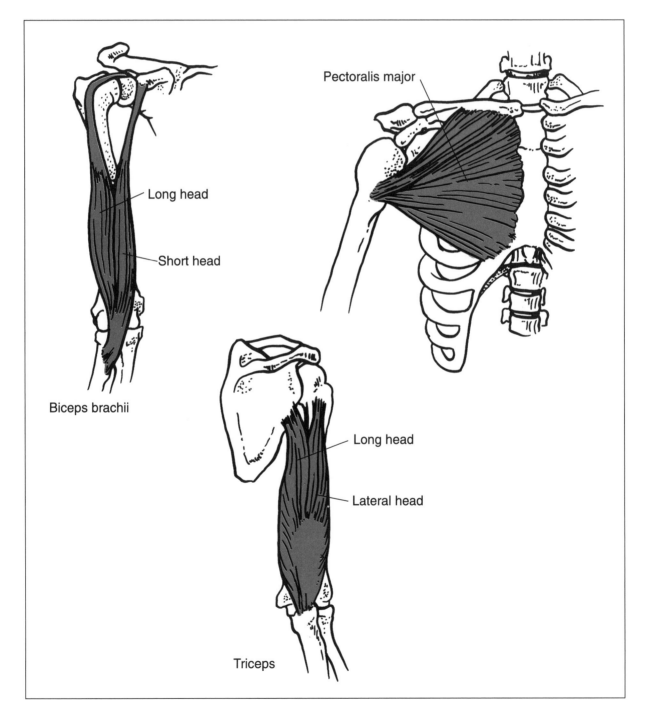

		Origin	Insertion	Action
Pectoralis, Biceps, and Triceps	Pectoralis major	Clavicular head: medial half of anterior aspect of clavicle Sternal head: sternum and cartilage of the 6 upper ribs	Lateral lip of bicipital groove of the humerus	Both heads: adduction, horizontal adduction and medial rotation of the humerus Clavicular head: flexion of humerus Sternal head: extension of humerus from a flexed position
	Biceps brachii	Long head: tubercle on superior aspect of glenoid cavity Short head: coracoid process	Radial tuberosity and bicipital aponeurosis	Elbow and shoulder flexion Supination of forearm Long head assists abduction Short head assists adduction Helps stabilize humerus in glenoid fossa during heavy lifting or carrying
	Triceps brachii	Long head: infra-glenoid tubercle of scapula Lateral head: postero-lateral surface of proximal humerus Medial head: lower 2/3 of posteromedial humerus	Olecranon process of ulna	Extension of elbow Long head only: extension of humerus

Functional Assessment

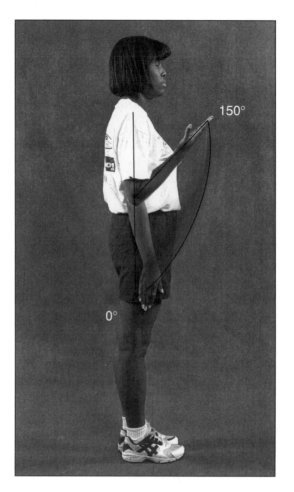

Figure 5.6 Normal flexion-extension of the elbow.

Normal range of motion at the elbow (figure 5.6):

Flexion = 150°

Extension = 0°

Elbow flexion may be limited by the muscle mass of the anterior arm or by a hypertonic triceps. Generally, the stretcher should be able to touch the front of her shoulder. Extension of the elbow may be limited by a hypertonic biceps. The triceps also acts to extend the humerus and may act to limit full flexion of the humerus if it is hypertonic.

Pectoralis Major Stretch—Prone

Stretching the pectoralis major can improve range of motion in **horizontal abduction**, flexion, extension, and external rotation of the humerus, depending on which fibers of the muscle are emphasized during the stretch.

1. The stretcher is prone, with his face resting in the face cradle, or his head turned to one side if no face cradle is available. His right arm is abducted to 90 degrees and externally rotated, with the elbow bent to 90 degrees. His upper arm rests on the table. Stand at the right side of the table and ask the stretcher to lift his right arm toward the ceiling as high as possible, keeping the forearm horizontal. As he lifts, make sure he does not lift his sternum off the table, which would indicate that he is rotating his trunk. This starting position lengthens the right pectoralis major to its pain-free end range.

By changing the angle of abduction of the arm, you can emphasize different fibers of the pectoralis major. Less abduction (45 degrees) focuses on the clavicular head; more abduction (135 degrees) focuses more on the lower fibers of the sterno-costal head.

2. Support the stretcher's right arm from the elbow to the hand using your right forearm and hand (figure 5.7). Ask the stretcher to begin slowly to attempt to bring his arm down and across his chest, leading with the elbow, isometrically contracting the pectoralis major.

3. After the isometric push, the stretcher relaxes and breathes in. During this time, maintain the arm in the starting position.

4. On the exhale, ask the stretcher to lift his arm higher, keeping the forearm horizontal and his sternum to the table.

5. Repeat 2 to 3 times.

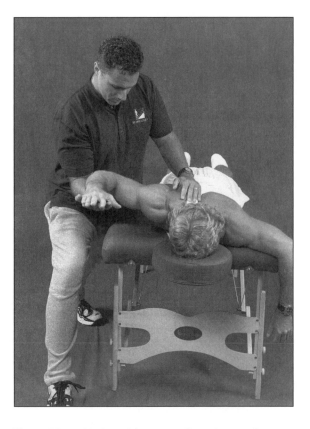

Figure 5.7 Initiation of the pectoralis major stretch, prone. Be sure the stretcher does not lift his sternum off the table.

Pectoralis Major Self-Stretch

Self-stretching of the pectoralis can be done using a doorway to provide resistance during the isometric phase (figure 5.8). Raise your arm higher or lower to stretch different parts of the pectoralis. Be aware of your posture, and use a wide front-to-back stance, keeping your back lengthened and not arched.

Biceps Stretch—Supine

This stretch is for improving the range of elbow and shoulder extension.

1. The stretcher lies supine with his right shoulder at the edge of the table. His right elbow is straight, and his shoulder is extended as far as possible. His forearm is in neutral, neither supinated nor pronated (the palm faces inward). This position lengthens the bicep to its end range.

2. Offer resistance to the isometric contraction of the biceps by placing your left hand against his right forearm. Use your right hand to stabilize his shoulder (figure 5.9).

3. Direct the stretcher to begin slowly to attempt to flex his right shoulder and elbow, isometrically contracting the biceps brachii. ("Try to bring your hand toward the ceiling.")

4. After the isometric push, the stretcher relaxes and inhales deeply. During this time, the arm may drop toward the floor or be maintained in the starting position.

5. On the exhale, the stretcher contracts the triceps to extend the arm farther, deepening the biceps stretch.

6. Repeat 2 to 3 times.

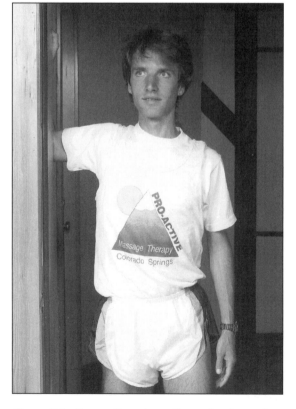

Figure 5.8 Pectoralis major self-stretch using a door-jamb.

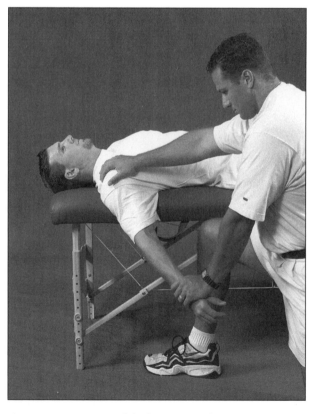

Figure 5.9 Initiation of the biceps stretch, supine.

Biceps Self-Stretch

This can be an awkward muscle to self-stretch, but it can be done. Find a horizontal surface, like a railing, a dance barre, or the back of a chair. You can also use the doorknob on a closed door. Stand (or kneel) with your arm straight, palm facing inward, and extend your arm behind you as far as you can, keeping your torso upright. Rest your forearm on your horizontal object or grasp the doorknob. From this starting position, try to push your hand toward the floor (flexion of the shoulder and elbow), isometrically contracting the biceps. After the isometric phase, extend your arm back farther. You may need to kneel down to properly position yourself for this stretch (figure 5.10).

Triceps Stretch—Prone

This stretch is used to improve flexion at the shoulder with the elbow bent.

1. The stretcher is prone, with his head resting in the face cradle or turned to the side. He flexes his right shoulder and elbow to place his right hand on his right scapula (figure 5.11). He keeps his arm as close to his ear as possible. This lengthens the triceps to its end range.

2. Place your hand against the stretcher's posterior elbow and ask him to begin to push slowly against you, attempting to bring his elbow toward the floor, isometrically contracting the triceps.

3. After the isometric push, the stretcher relaxes and breathes in. During this time, maintain the arm in the starting position.

4. On the exhale, ask the stretcher to reach farther down his back, keeping his arm close to his ear, deepening the triceps stretch.

5. Repeat the sequence 2 to 3 more times.

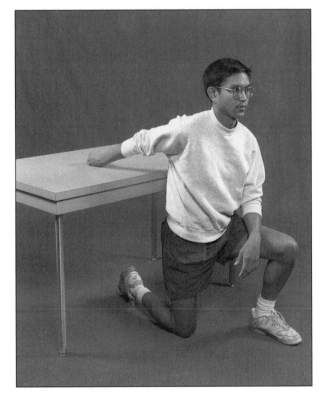

Figure 5.10 Biceps self-stretch.

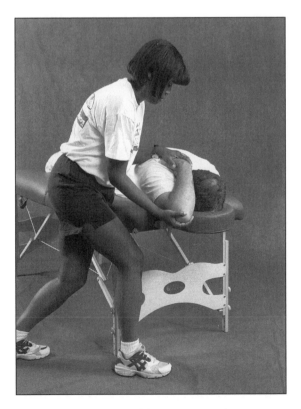

Figure 5.11 Initiation of the triceps stretch, prone.

Triceps Self-Stretch

For self-stretching, a seated position works the best because it helps keep you from arching your back, although it can be done standing. You can provide isometric resistance for this stretch by using your other arm and hand (figure 5.12). Be sure to maintain length in the spine (low back and neck) during this stretch to achieve the best results.

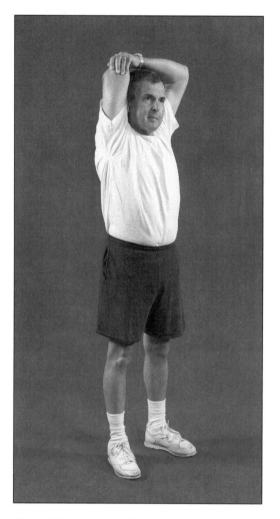

Figure 5.12 Triceps self-stretch. Use good posture.

WRIST FLEXORS AND EXTENSORS
Anatomy

Baseball players, racquetball players, musicians, grocery clerks, and typists are commonly afflicted with hypertonic wrist and forearm muscles. Maintaining good range of motion at the wrist can help reduce the risk of overuse tendinitis or repetitive stress injuries like carpal tunnel syndrome.

Limited range of motion at the wrist is uncommon unless the wrist has been immobilized for some reason. Because the wrist muscles are used extensively in daily activity, even "leg-sport" athletes will appreciate stretching these muscles.

Three primary muscles act to flex the wrist: flexor carpi radialis, flexor carpi ulnaris, and palmaris longus. Their common origin on the medial epicondyle is the site of "golfer's elbow," an overuse tendinitis.

Like the flexors of the wrist, three primary muscles extend the wrist: extensor carpi radialis longus, extensor carpi radialis brevis, and extensor carpi ulnaris. Their common origin on the lateral epicondyle is the primary site of "tennis elbow," an overuse tendinitis common in racket sports.

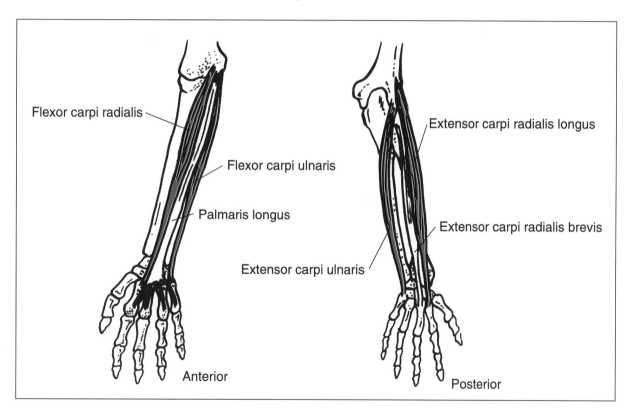

		Origin	Insertion	Action
Wrist Flexors	Carpi radialis	Medial epicondyle of humerus	Base of 2nd and 3rd metacarpals	Flexion and abduction of wrist
	Carpi ulnaris	Medial epicondyle of humerus and proximal posterior ulna	Pisiform, hamate and base of 5th metacarpal	Flexion and adduction of wrist
	Palmaris longus (sometimes absent)	Medial epicondyle of humerus	Palmar aponeurosis	Assists flexion of wrist
Wrist Extensors	Carpi radialis longus	Lateral epicondyle and lateral supracondylar ridge of humerus	Base of 2nd metacarpal	Extension and abduction of wrist
	Carpi radialis brevis	Lateral epicondyle of humerus	Base of 3rd metacarpal	Extension of wrist
	Carpi ulnaris	Lateral epicondyle of humerus and proximal posterior ulna	Base of 5th metacarpal	Extension and adduction of wrist

Functional Assessment

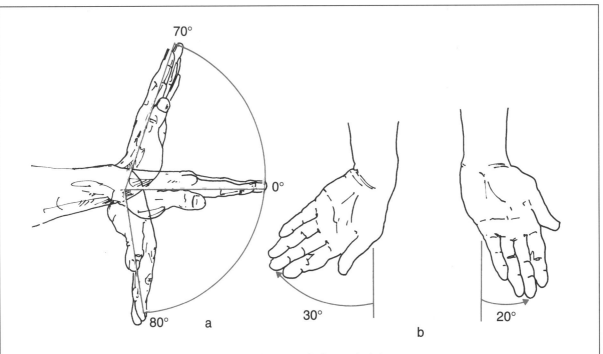

Figure 5.13   (a) Normal wrist flexion-extension. (b) Normal ulnar-radial deviation.

Normal range of motion, measured from the wrist in neutral (figure 5.13):

Flexion = 80°

Extension = 70°

Ulnar deviation (adduction) = 30°

Radial deviation (abduction) = 20°

Wrist Flexor Stretch—Supine

This stretch is used for increasing extension at the wrist.

1. The stretcher is supine, with her right elbow straight and her wrist and fingers extended as far as possible. This lengthens the right wrist (and finger) flexors to their pain-free end range.

2. Place the palm and fingers of your left hand over the palm and fingers of the stretcher's right hand, matching thumb to thumb and finger to finger. Your other hand stabilizes the stretcher's wrist and forearm (figure 5.14).

3. Direct the stretcher to start slowly to try to flex the wrist and fingers (including the thumb), isometrically contracting the flexors.

4. After the isometric push, the stretcher relaxes and breathes in. During this time, maintain her wrist and fingers in the starting position.

5. On the exhale, the stretcher contracts the wrist and finger extensors, deepening the wrist flexor stretch.

You may gently assist to deepen the stretch by pushing on the stretcher's fingers.

6. Repeat 2 to 3 times.

Wrist Extensor Stretch—Supine

This stretch is used for increasing wrist and finger flexion.

1. The stretcher is supine, with her right elbow straight and her wrist and fingers flexed as far as possible. This lengthens the right wrist (and finger) extensors to their pain-free end range. (The stretcher should fully flex her wrist first, and then curl her fingers as far as possible. If she makes a fist first, this limits her wrist flexion, which we want to optimize.)

2. Wrap your right hand over the stretcher's fist, matching thumb to thumb and finger to finger. Your other hand stabilizes the stretcher's wrist and forearm (figure 5.15).

3. Direct the stretcher to start slowly to try to extend the wrist and fingers (including the thumb), isometrically contracting the extensors.

4. After the isometric push, the stretcher relaxes and breathes in. During this time, maintain her wrist and fingers in the starting position.

5. On the exhale, the stretcher contracts the wrist and finger flexors to deepen the flexor stretch. You may gently assist to deepen the stretch by pushing on the stretcher's fingers.

6. Repeat 2 to 3 times.

Wrist Self-Stretch

You can easily provide isometric resistance for these stretches by using your other hand (figure 5.16).

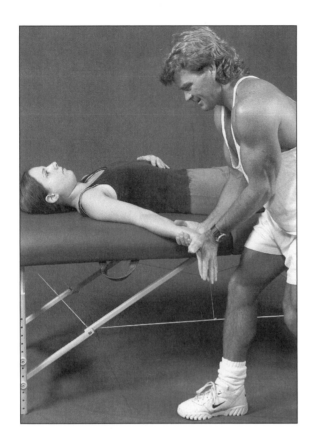

Figure 5.14   Initiation of the wrist flexor stretch.

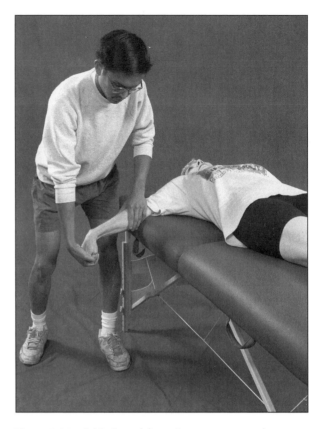

Figure 5.15   Initiation of the wrist extensor stretch.

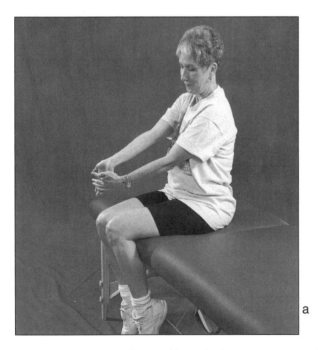

a

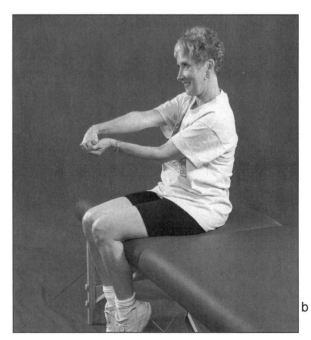

b

Figure 5.16   (a) Wrist flexor self-stretch. (b) Wrist extensor self-stretch.

Spiral Patterns for the Upper Extremity

The spiral-diagonal patterns for the arms are extremely useful for increasing range of motion in the shoulder girdle. They're also helpful in determining which muscles in a pattern of motion are weak or not firing properly. These individual muscles can then be isolated for single muscle stretching and/or strengthening.

Working with the upper extremity can seem complicated because we have the option of working with the elbow bent or straight in the two patterns that involve adduction (D1 flexion and D2 extension). The instructions are given assuming the elbow remains straight. As you gain more experience, you can work with the elbow bent and add resisted elbow extension during the isometric phase.

D1 Extension (Reverse Push-ups) Stretch

This stretch is for increasing range of motion in flexion, adduction, and external rotation.

1. The stretcher is supine, with her right shoulder in as much flexion, adduction, and external rotation as possible. The stretcher keeps her elbow straight and both shoulder blades on the table. Her forearm is supinated, and her wrist and fingers are flexed. To gain as much adduction and flexion as possible, have the stretcher turn her head to the left so her chin does not interfere with her arm motion. This position lengthens the target muscles to their end range. These include the infraspinatus, middle trapezius, rhomboids, teres minor, posterior deltoid, and pronator teres.

2. Stand at the head of the table to support and stabilize the arm and wrist (figure 5.17). Remember, your hand contacts give the stretcher proprioceptive cues about which way to push or pull. Your hand positions should match your verbal commands.

3. Direct the stretcher to begin slowly to try to initiate the D1 extension pattern, beginning with pronation and internal rotation, then abduction, then extension. ("Begin by rotating, then push down and out.")

4. After the isometric push, the stretcher relaxes and inhales deeply. As she relaxes, maintain the arm in the starting position.

5. On the exhale, the stretcher moves the arm farther into flexion, then into adduction, and then into external rotation and supination. Remember, we want a blend of all three directions to keep moving in a diagonal line. Be sure she keeps her shoulder blades on the table so the stretch comes as she reaches from the shoulder joint.

Support the arm but do not push to deepen the stretch.

6. Repeat 2 to 3 times.

D1 Flexion (Self-Feeding) Stretch

This stretch is used to improve range of motion in extension, abduction, and internal rotation.

1. The stretcher lies supine at the edge of the table. She has her right shoulder in extension, abduction, and internal rotation as far as possible. Her forearm is pronated, with her wrist and fingers extended. This position lengthens the target muscles to their end range. These include the pectorals (clavicular head), anterior deltoid, coracobrachialis, biceps brachii, infraspinatus, and supinator.

2. Support and stabilize the arm and wrist (figure 5.18). Remember, your hand contacts give the stretcher proprioceptive cues about which way to push or pull. Your hand positions should match your verbal commands.

3. Direct the stretcher to begin slowly to try to initiate the D1 flexion pattern, beginning with external rotation, then adduction, then flexion. ("Begin by rotating, then push up and across your body.") The stretcher is not attempting to bend her elbow.

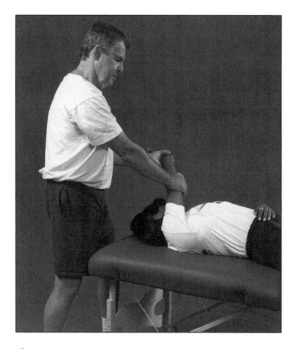

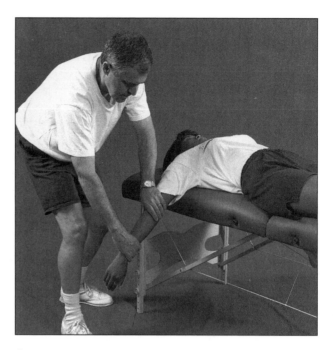

Figure 5.17 Initiation of D1 extension. The shoulder is flexed, adducted, and externally rotated; the forearm is supinated and the wrist and fingers flexed.

Figure 5.18 Initiation of D1 flexion. The shoulder is extended, abducted, and internally rotated; the forearm is pronated, and the wrist and fingers extended.

4. After the isometric push, the stretcher relaxes and inhales deeply. As she relaxes, maintain the arm in the starting position.

5. On the exhale, the stretcher moves the arm farther, into extension, then into abduction, and then internal rotation and pronation. Remember, we want a blend of all three directions to keep moving in a diagonal line.

Again, support the arm but do not push to deepen the stretch.

6. Repeat 2 to 3 times.

D2 Flexion (Drawing a Sword) Stretch

This stretch is used to improve range of motion in extension, adduction, and internal rotation.

1. The stretcher is prone, with her right shoulder extended, adducted, and internally rotated. The forearm is pronated, with the wrist and fingers flexed. This is a modified "hammerlock" position, with the elbow straight and the thumb pointing away from her back. This position lengthens the target muscles to their end range. These include the anterior deltoid, coracobrachialis, pectorals, and biceps brachii.

2. Support and stabilize the arm and wrist (figure 5.19). Remember, your hand contacts give the stretcher proprioceptive cues about which way to push or pull; your hand positions should match your verbal commands.

3. Direct the stretcher to begin slowly to try to initiate the D2 flexion pattern, beginning with supination and external rotation, then abduction, then flexion. ("Begin by rotating, then push through and away from your body.")

4. After the isometric push, the stretcher relaxes and inhales deeply. As she relaxes, maintain the arm in the starting position.

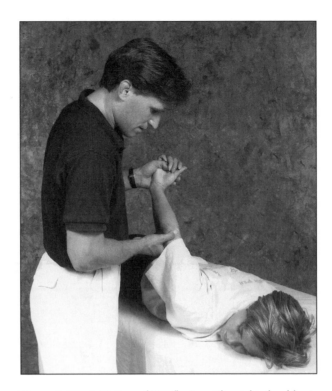

Figure 5.19 Initiation of D2 flexion. The right shoulder is extended, adducted, and internally rotated; the forearm is pronated, and the wrist and fingers flexed.

5. On the exhale, the stretcher moves her arm farther into extension, then into adduction, and then internal rotation and pronation. Remember, we want a blend of all three directions to keep moving in a diagonal line.

As before, support the arm but do not push to deepen the stretch.

6. Repeat 2 to 3 times.

D2 Extension (Sheathing a Sword) Stretch

This stretch is for improving range of motion in flexion, abduction, and external rotation.

1. The stretcher lies supine, with her right shoulder flexed, abducted, and externally rotated as far as possible. Her forearm is supinated, with the wrist and fingers extended. This is the starting position for D2 extension and lengthens the target muscles to their end range. These include the pectorals (sternal head), anterior deltoid, subscapularis, biceps brachii, pronator teres, latissimus dorsi, and teres major.

2. Support and stabilize the arm and wrist (figure 5.20). Remember, your hand contacts give the stretcher proprioceptive cues about which way to push or pull; your hand positions should match your verbal commands.

3. Direct the stretcher to begin slowly to try to initiate the D2 extension pattern, beginning with internal rotation, then adduction, then extension. ("Begin by rotating, then push toward the ceiling and across your body.") The stretcher is not trying to bend her elbow.

4. After the isometric push, the stretcher relaxes and inhales deeply. As she relaxes, maintain the arm in the starting position.

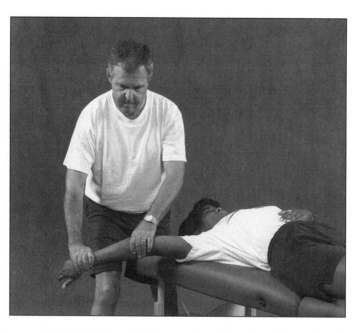

Figure 5.20 Initiation of D2 extension. The shoulder is flexed, abducted, and externally rotated; the forearm is supinated, and the wrist and fingers extended.

5. On the exhale, the stretcher moves her arm farther into flexion, then into abduction, and then external rotation and supination. Remember, we want a blend of all three directions to keep moving in a diagonal line.

Again, support the arm but do not push to deepen the stretch.

6. Repeat 2 to 3 times.

Chapter 6

Stretches for the Torso and Neck

This chapter addresses the muscles of the torso and neck. This is a somewhat arbitrary division because some of the muscles in this chapter also contribute to motion of the arms and legs. The muscles covered in this section are primarily postural muscles. Almost everyone has excess tension in these muscles, so facilitated stretching techniques are a quick and simple way to provide more ease and comfort in these core areas. The nature of our daily lives requires a great deal of flexion in the torso and neck—we sit at desks, in cars, in front of the television. Our chairs are not really designed to support our bodies well, and the postural muscles are called upon to literally "take up the slack." Most sports also require a great deal of support and active involvement from these muscles. The following stretches can be used as preventive techniques or to help relieve pain caused by imbalance in these muscles.

CERVICAL AREA
Anatomy

The cervical, or neck, area is a storehouse of muscular tension. Many people experience discomfort or pain in this region because of postural stress, job-related activities, or trauma. Stretching these muscles can provide great relief from tightness and pain but can also create pain if done too aggressively. When performing these stretches,

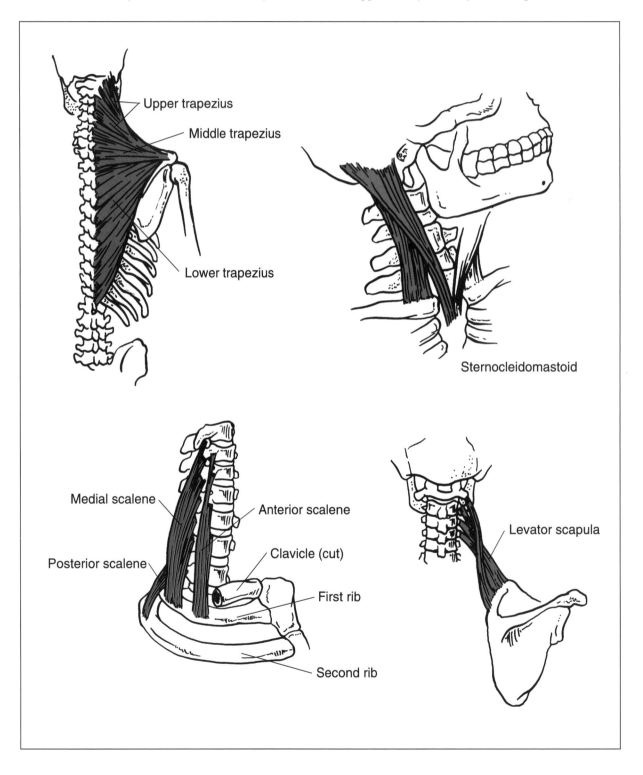

be especially careful that the stretcher is pain free at all times. If you are working with a stretcher who has suffered any type of neck injury, work cautiously. Sometimes the stretcher may not realize that he is overworking and will end up with increased pain a day or two after stretching.

Muscles of the cervical region include the upper trapezius, sternocleidomastoid (SCM), scalenes, and levator scapula. We discuss each here, then describe the functional assessment of the cervical spine.

▼ Many people have upper traps that are hypertonic. When the upper traps are too tight, they can cause headaches and pain. They also develop significant trigger points.

▼ The sternocleidomastoid is a complex muscle with many actions. At its inferior attachments, it has two parts, the sternal and clavicular. These two divisions merge into a common attachment on the skull.

▼ The scalene muscles are divided into three sections: anterior, middle, and posterior. They are strongly implicated in thoracic outlet syndrome, carpal tunnel syndrome, and other painful conditions of the neck, shoulder, and arm. This is because the brachial plexus (a bundle of nerves) and the subclavian artery pass between the anterior and middle scalenes and may become entrapped if the muscles are hypertonic.

The levator scapula is often implicated in complaints of neck stiffness, especially when rotation is limited. Postural stress causes this muscle to be hypertonic.

CERVICAL AREA

		Origin	Insertion	Action
Trapezius	Upper trapezius	Occiput Spinous processes of C7-T12 and the ligamentum nuchae	Posterior aspect of lateral 1/3 of the clavicle	Unilaterally: elevation of shoulder, lateral flexion of head and neck Bilaterally: extension of head and neck
Sternocleidomastoid	Sternocleidomastoid	Sternal division: anterior aspect of manubrium of sternum Clavicular division: anterior, superior aspect of medial 1/3 of the clavicle	Lateral aspect of mastoid process Lateral half of superior nuchal line on the occipital bone	Bilaterally: flexion of head and neck, especially against resistance of gravity Unilaterally: rotation of head to opposite side, assists lateral flexion to same side
Scalenes	Anterior scalene	Anterior aspect of tranverse processes of C3–C6	Superior aspect of 1st rib	Lateral flexion of cervical spine Assists neck flexion Elevates ribs during inspiration
	Middle scalene	Transverse processes of C2–C7	Superior aspect of the 1st rib lateral to anterior scalene	Lateral flexion of cervical spine Elevates ribs during inspiration
	Posterior scalene	Transverse processes of C5–C7	Superior aspect of the 2nd rib posterior to middle scalene	Lateral flexion of cervical spine Elevates ribs during inspiration
Levator Scapula	Levator scapula	Transverse processes of C1–C4	Superior angle and medial border of scapula	Bilaterally: extends head and neck, assists shoulder shrugs Unilaterally: assists downward rotation and elevation of scapula, assists lateral flexion and rotation of neck to same side

Functional Assessment

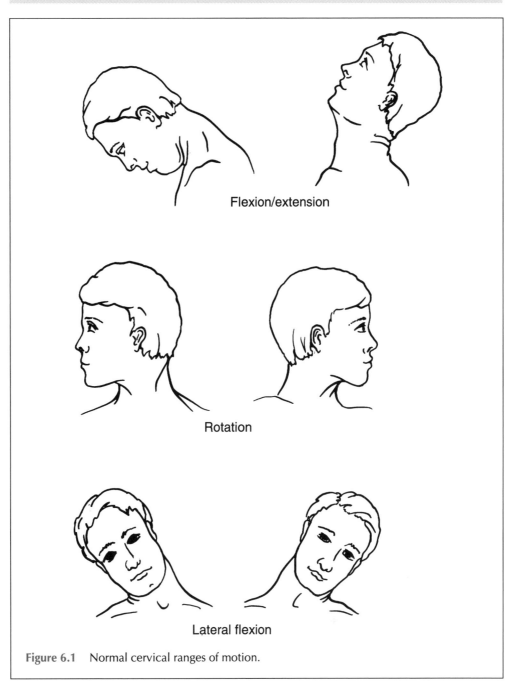

Flexion/extension

Rotation

Lateral flexion

Figure 6.1 Normal cervical ranges of motion.

The neck is capable of motion in six directions: flexion, extension, lateral flexion to each side, and rotation to each side (figure 6.1). These motions can also be combined to create a greater variety of movement.

Movement of the head and neck is more complex than movements around other joints. Many muscles contribute to each movement, and it is difficult to isolate one muscle at a time. Therefore, even though our focus is on four major groups (upper trapezius, sternocleidomastoid (SCM), scalenes, and levator scapula), smaller muscles that contribute to the same motion will also be affected.

Range of motion for the head and neck is as follows:

Flexion = 85°

Extension = 70°

Rotation = 80°

Lateral flexion = 40°

Upper Trapezius Stretch—Supine

This stretch is used to improve range of motion in cervical rotation and flexion and shoulder depression.

1. The stretcher is supine. Help him rotate his head to the right as far as possible without pain, then tuck his chin as far as possible. If the right shoulder interferes with this motion, have the stretcher pull it down, away from the head. The stretcher also pulls his left shoulder down away from his head. This starting position lengthens the left upper trap to its pain-free end range.

2. Place your left hand at the stretcher's occiput, fingers pointing toward the ceiling. Place your right hand on his left shoulder (figure 6.2). Ask the stretcher to begin slowly to push against both of your hands, as if bringing the back of his head and his left shoulder together. You provide matching resistance for this isometric contraction, being sure that the client is pushing equally from both ends and breathing normally throughout.

3. After the isometric push, the stretcher relaxes and breathes in. As he relaxes, maintain the head in the starting position.

4. On the exhale, the stretcher rotates his head farther to the right, tucks his chin more (if possible), and pulls his left shoulder farther away from his head. This deepens the upper trapezius stretch.

5. Repeat 2 to 3 times.

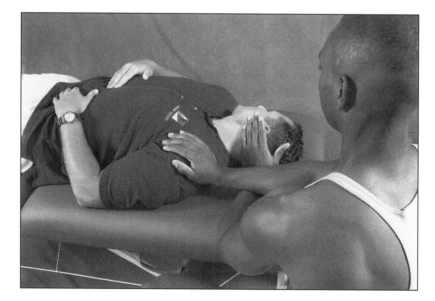

Figure 6.2 Initiation of upper trapezius stretch, supine.

Upper Trapezius Self-Stretch—Supine

This is an easy stretch to do by yourself. Lie down on your back, keep your neck lengthened, and turn your head to the right as far as possible; tuck your chin as far as possible, and pull your left shoulder toward your feet. Now, place your left arm under your body to anchor your left shoulder. Wrap your right arm around your head so that your right fingers can hold the base of your skull (figure 6.3).

From this starting position, try to bring your left shoulder and the back of your head toward each other. Following this isometric contraction of the left upper traps, increase their stretch by turning farther to the right, tucking your chin, and pulling your left shoulder farther away from your head.

Sternocleidomastoid (SCM) Stretch—Supine

This stretch is used to improve rotation of the head and neck.

1. The stretcher is supine. Keeping his neck lengthened, help him rotate his head to the right as far as possible without pain. This starting position lengthens the right SCM to its pain-free end range.

2. Cradle the stretcher's head in your right hand; place your left hand just above his left ear (figure 6.4). Ask the client to begin slowly to attempt to rotate his head to the left. He is not trying to lift his head from the table. You provide matching resistance for this isometric contraction, being sure that the client is breathing normally throughout.

3. After the isometric push, the stretcher relaxes and breathes in. As he relaxes, maintain the head in the starting position.

4. On the exhale, the stretcher rotates his head farther to the right, deepening the stretch on the right SCM.

5. Repeat 2 to 3 times.

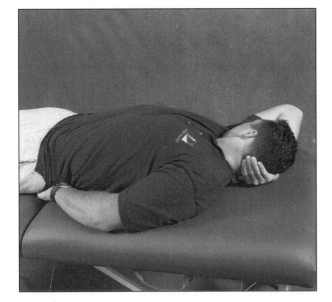

Figure 6.3   Upper trapezius self-stretch.

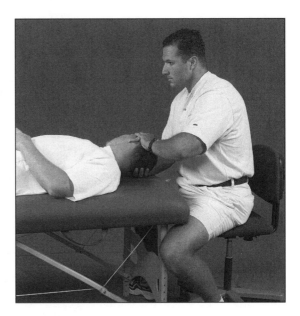

Figure 6.4   Initiation of SCM stretch, supine.

Sternocleidomastoid (SCM) Self-Stretch—Supine

Lie down on your back and turn your head to the right as far as possible, keeping your neck lengthened. Use your right hand to resist your attempt to turn your head back to the left. Be sure not to try to lift your head from the floor, but only turn to the left (figure 6.5). After this isometric contraction of the SCM, increase the stretch by turning farther to the right.

Scalene Stretch—Supine

This stretch is for improving lateral flexion of the head and neck.

1. The stretcher is supine. Help him laterally flex his head and neck to the left as far as possible without pain. Prevent him from adding rotation to the motion by asking him to keep his nose pointed directly at the ceiling. He also pulls his right shoulder away from his head. This starting position lengthens the right scalenes to their pain-free end range.

2. Place your left hand on his head just above his right ear. Place your right hand against his right shoulder to anchor it in place (figure 6.6). Direct the stretcher to begin slowly to push against your left hand, as if he is trying to bring his right ear directly to his right shoulder. Be sure he does not add rotation to his effort. He does not push up with his shoulder because we're using the shoulder to anchor the ribs, which are the distal attachment of the scalenes. You provide matching resistance for this isometric contraction, being sure that the stretcher is breathing normally throughout.

3. After the isometric push, the stretcher relaxes and breathes in. As he relaxes, maintain the head in the starting position.

4. On the exhale, ask the stretcher to bring his left ear closer to his left shoulder, being sure to keep his nose pointed directly at the ceiling. This deepens the stretch of the right scalenes.

5. Repeat 2 to 3 times, then help the stretcher reposition his head to do the same stretch for the left scalenes.

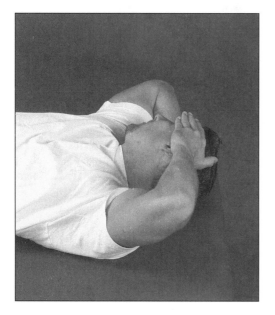

Figure 6.5 SCM self-stretch. Be sure not to try to lift your head from the table.

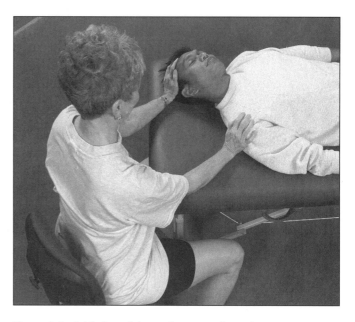

Figure 6.6 Initiation of the scalene stretch, supine.

6. For more specificity, you can isolate the anterior or posterior scalenes by rotating the head as follows:

Left anterior scalene—laterally flex the neck to the right, then rotate the head 45 degrees to the left. From this position, follow the stretching sequence (figure 6.7a).

Left posterior scalene—laterally flex the neck to the right, then rotate the head 45 degrees to the right. From this position, follow the stretching sequence (figure 6.7b).

Right anterior scalene—laterally flex the neck to the left, then rotate the head 45 degrees to the right. From this position, follow the stretching sequence (figure 6.7c).

Right posterior scalene—laterally flex the neck to the left, then rotate the head 45 degrees to the left. From this position, follow the stretching sequence (figure 6.7d).

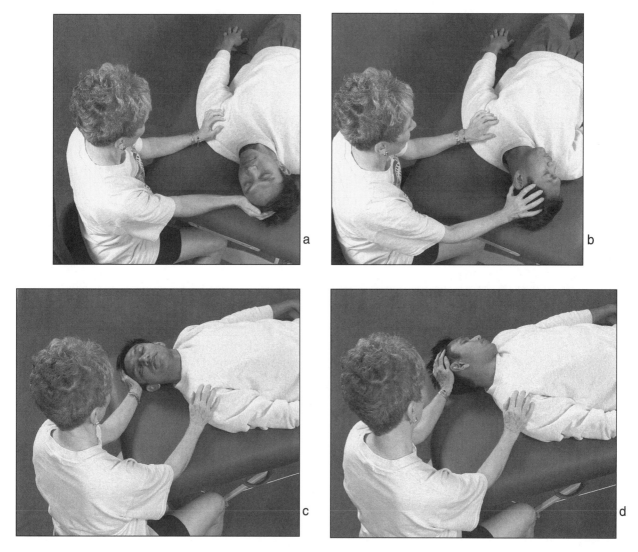

Figure 6.7 Isolating the scalenes. (a) Left anterior scalene. (b) Left posterior scalene. (c) Right anterior scalene. (d) Right posterior scalene.

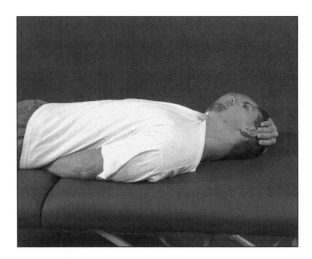

Figure 6.8 Scalene self-stretch.

Scalene Self-Stretch—Supine

Lie down on your back. Pull your left shoulder away from your ear and anchor it by placing your left arm under your body. Keeping your nose pointed toward the ceiling (so you don't rotate your head), laterally flex your neck to bring your right ear as close to your right shoulder as possible. Bring your right arm up around your head, with your fingers holding just above your left ear (figure 6.8). Now, try to bring your left ear toward your left shoulder. Don't try to lift your head from the floor, and keep your nose pointed at the ceiling. After this isometric contraction of the left scalenes, see if you can bring your right ear closer to your right shoulder. Don't pull it with your hand; use your neck muscles. You may need to lift your head slightly if it won't slide on the floor.

Levator Scapula Stretch—Supine

This stretch helps improve head and neck flexion.

1. The stretcher is supine. Point out the origin, insertion, and path of the left levator scapula to him. Standing at his head, place your left hand against the superior angle of his left scapula and push it away from his head. Stabilize your left arm against your left hip, being aware of your posture. This fixes the scapular attachment of the levator. With your right hand holding at the occiput, help the client flex his head and neck to touch his chin to his chest. From this position, rotate the head approximately 45 degrees to the right to fully lengthen the left levator scapula. This is an approximate starting position because some stretchers may not feel the stretch here. You will need to play with the positioning until the stretcher can feel the stretch along the path of the levator. This is the pain-free end range. Once you've found the right position, you may find it more comfortable to use the back of your right hand or your torso to support his head.

2. From this position, direct the stretcher to begin slowly pushing his head and neck back toward the left corner of the table. You provide matching resistance for this isometric contraction, being sure that the client is breathing normally throughout (figure 6.9).

3. After the isometric push, the stretcher relaxes and breathes in. As he relaxes, maintain the head in the starting position.

4. On the exhale, ask the client to flex his head and neck to bring his chin closer to his chest. Maintain the rotational component. This increases the stretch of the left levator scapula.

5. Repeat 2 to 3 times, then help the client reposition his head to do the same stretch for the right levator scapula.

Levator Scapula Self-Stretch—Sitting

Sit comfortably, keeping your spine lengthened. Drop your head to your chest, then turn your chin to the right about 45 degrees. Bring your right hand up to the top of your head and pull slightly until you feel a stretch of the left levator scapula. You may need to play with your head position a little to find this place of stretch. Be sure to keep your spine long (figure 6.10). Following this isometric contraction of the levator scapula, increase the stretch by tucking your chin more.

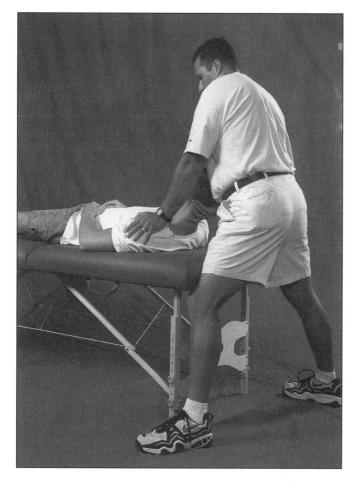

Figure 6.9   Initiation of the levator scapula stretch.

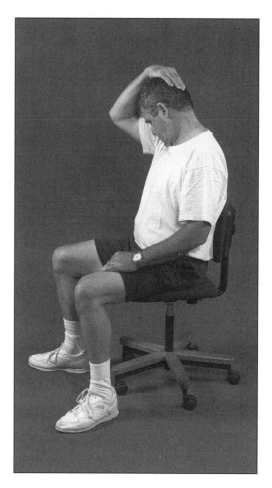

Figure 6.10   Levator scapula self-stretch.

THORACIC AND LUMBAR AREA
Anatomy

The thoracic and lumbar areas often maintain chronic muscular tension, which can be greatly alleviated through effective stretching. Many people experience pain in these areas from trauma, job-related injury, and/or postural stress. When performing these stretches, be especially aware that the stretcher is working in the pain-free zone at all

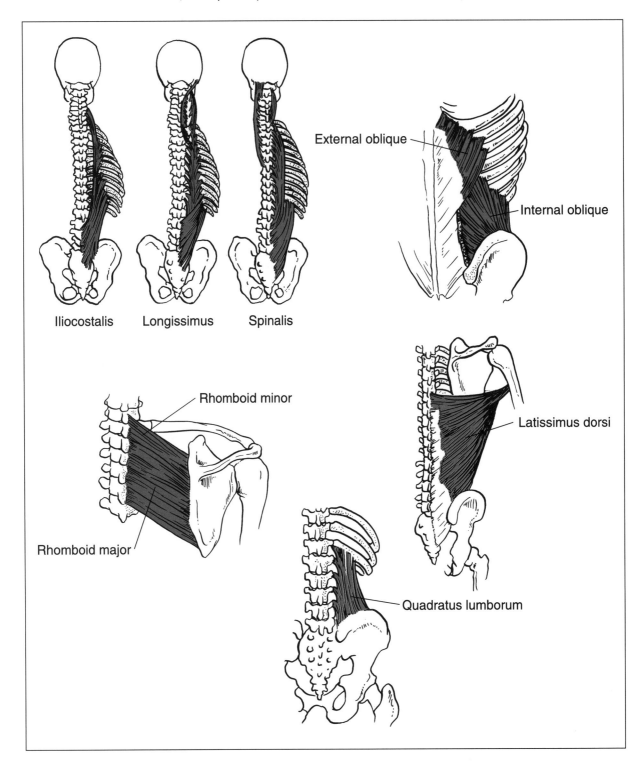

Iliocostalis   Longissimus   Spinalis

External oblique

Internal oblique

Rhomboid minor

Rhomboid major

Latissimus dorsi

Quadratus lumborum

times. If you are working with a stretcher who has suffered any type of back injury, work cautiously. Sometimes, the stretcher may not realize he is overworking and will have increased pain a day or two after stretching.

The back extensors, trunk rotators, rhomboids, quadratus lumborum, and latissimus dorsi support the thoracic and lumbar spine.

The *back extensors* consist of the erector spinae group (iliocostalis, longissimus, and spinalis, each with 2 or 3 divisions) and the transversospinalis group (semispinalis thoracis, multifidus, rotatores, interspinales, and intertransversarii). We illustrate the erector spinae here but are not listing the origins and insertions. These muscles, acting bilaterally, extend the spine. Acting unilaterally, they assist trunk rotation. When they are hypertonic, they can create back pain and limit spinal flexion and rotation. They are also common sites for trigger points.

Trunk rotation involves the thoracic and lumbar spine. The major muscles of rotation are the internal and external oblique abdominals, assisted by the erector spinae, semispinalis thoracis, multifidus, and rotatores. We are listing only the oblique abdominals here. The external oblique angles downward and medially from the ribs. The internal oblique angles upward and medially from the lateral and posterior iliac crest.

Although the *rhomboids* often are tender to palpation, they are commonly overstretched rather than hypertonic. This overstretched condition is likely in people with rounded shoulders, where the pectoralis muscles draw the shoulders forward. In such a situation, stretching the pectorals and strengthening the rhomboids would be indicated.

The *quadratus lumborum* (QL) is an important component of a strong and healthy low back. When this muscle is hypertonic, it develops trigger points that refer pain to the hips, gluteal area, and down the leg. The QL is always involved in low back pain, even that which results from disk problems or misalignment of the lumbar vertebrae.

Latissimus dorsi forms part of the posterior axillary border and is used in many activities in which the arm moves from overhead downward, like chopping wood, swimming, and rock climbing. It's often overlooked as a source of back pain.

		Origin	Insertion	Action
Oblique Abdominals	External oblique	Lateral and inferior aspects of the lower 8 ribs	Anterior iliac crest and linea alba via the abdominal aponeurosis	Bilaterally: increase intra-abdominal pressure, trunk flexion Unilaterally: lateral flexion of trunk to same side, rotation of trunk to opposite side
	Internal oblique	Thoracolumbar fascia Anterior and lateral iliac crest Lateral half of inguinal ligament	Cartilage of the lower 3 ribs Linea alba via the abdominal aponeurosis	Bilaterally: increase intra-abdominal pressure, trunk flexion Unilaterally: lateral flexion and rotation of trunk to same side

(continued)

THORACIC AND LUMBAR AREA

		Origin	Insertion	Action
Rhomboids	Rhomboid major	Ligamentum nuchae and spinous processes of C7 and T1	Medial border of scapula, at root of spine	Adduct and elevate scapula Help stabilize scapula during arm movements
	Rhomboid minor	Spinous processes of T2–T5	Medial border of scapula, from its spine to its inferior angle	Adduct and elevate scapula Help stabilize scapula during arm movements
Quadratus Lumborum	Quadratus lumborum	Posterior iliac crest and iliolumbar ligament	Inferior border of the 12th rib and transverse processes of L1–L5	Bilaterally: stabilizes the 12th rib during respiration, assists extension of lumbar spine Unilaterally: lateral flexion of trunk or elevation of ilium
Latissimus Dorsi	Latissimus dorsi	Spinous processes of T7–L5 Sacrum via the lumbar aponeurosis Crest of ilium	Medial aspect of bicipital groove of humerus	Extension of arm from a flexed position Adduction Shoulder depression Assists internal rotation Provides a "vest pocket" for inferior angle of scapula, holding it against ribs

Functional Assessment

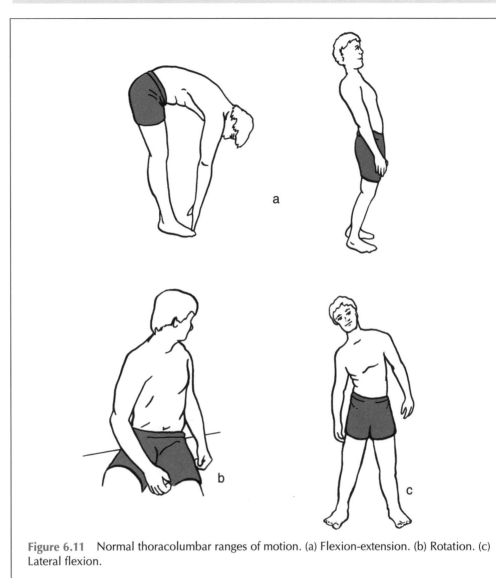

Figure 6.11   Normal thoracolumbar ranges of motion. (a) Flexion-extension. (b) Rotation. (c) Lateral flexion.

Trunk motion is a combination of movement at the lumbar and thoracic spine (figure 6.11). Six directions are possible: flexion, extension, rotation to each side, and lateral flexion to each side. These movements can also be combined to create a greater variety of motion.

Movement in the lumbar and thoracic spine is a complex combination of motion at each vertebra. Many muscles contribute to every motion, and it is difficult to isolate one muscle at a time. Therefore, even though our focus is on the major muscles of the trunk region, smaller muscles that contribute to the same motion will also be affected.

The thoracolumbar range of motion is as follows:

Flexion = 90°

Extension = 30°

Rotation = 45°

Lateral flexion = 30°

THORACIC AND LUMBAR AREA

Back Extensors Stretch—Seated

This stretch is used to improve trunk flexion.

1. The stretcher is seated at the edge of the treatment table (or on the floor), with her knees slightly bent (to relax the hamstrings) during this stretch. She leans forward as far as possible by contracting the rectus abdominis and psoas. The stretcher focuses on bending from the hips and not "stooping" in her upper back. She keeps her head in line with her spine or may drop her chin to her chest. This lengthens her back extensors to their pain-free end of range.

2. Place both hands on the stretcher's lower back to provide resistance to the isometric contraction of the back extensors (figure 6.12).

● 3. Direct the stretcher to begin slowly to attempt to extend her spine, isometrically contracting the back extensors. She focuses on the part of her spine where your hands are. The stretcher does not use her arms to push back.

4. After the isometric push, the stretcher relaxes and inhales deeply. During this time, maintain the spine in the starting position.

▨ 5. On the exhale, the stretcher contracts her rectus abdominis and psoas to bend farther forward, deepening the stretch of the back extensors. Remind the stretcher to keep her back lengthened and bend from the hips.

▲ 6. Repeat 3 to 5 times, each time moving your hands farther up the back (figure 6.13a). As your hands move up her back, she moves the focus of her isometric contraction to match. Once the focus of the isometric contraction has moved to the midback and upper

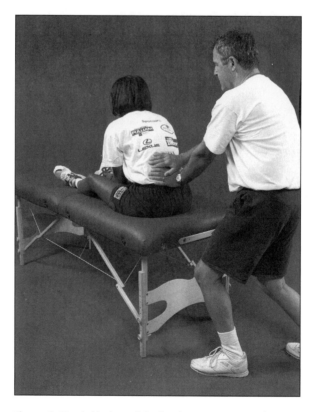

Figure 6.12 Initiation of the back extensors stretch.

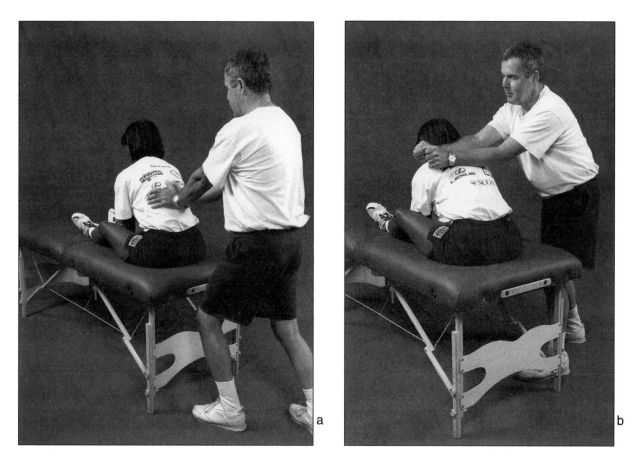

a   b

Figure 6.13 Moving up the back. Once the focus of the isometric contraction has moved to the midback and upper back, the stretcher may "stoop" and pull her chin to her chest during the stretching phase to fully lengthen the extensors of the midback and upper back area.

back, the stretcher may "stoop" and pull her chin to her chest during the stretching phase to fully lengthen the extensors of the midback and upper back area (figure 6.13b).

Back Extensors Self-Stretch—Seated

Sit in a chair and, keeping your upper back straight and bending from the hips, bend forward as far as you can (figure 6.14). Use a folded towel across your lower back to provide resistance during the isometric contraction of the extensors. Move the towel farther up your back with each round of stretching. As you work your way up to the midback and upper back, you may bend your upper back and pull your chin to your chest to increase the stretch of the midback and upper back extensors.

Trunk Rotators Stretch—Seated

Twisting to the right stretches the right external oblique and the left internal oblique.

1. The stretcher is seated on the table, with his knees bent and legs hanging over the side. This position stabilizes the hips. Keeping his spine lengthened and without arching his back, he twists to the right as far as he can, keeping his nose in alignment with his sternum (this neutral position is more comfortable). This position lengthens the left trunk rotators to their pain-free end range.

2. Reach under the stretcher's right arm to place your right hand on his anterior shoulder. Place your left hand on his left scapula, near the infero-medial border. Ask him

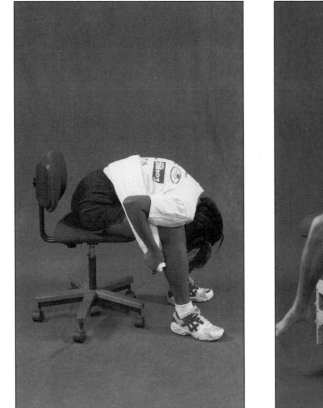

Figure 6.14   Back extensors self-stretch. Use a folded towel across your lower back to provide resistance.

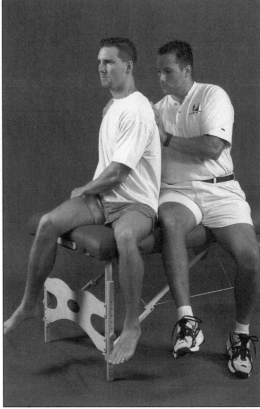

Figure 6.15   Initiation of the trunk rotators stretch.

to begin slowly to twist back to the left, keeping his head in neutral (figure 6.15). Be sure he is twisting from his trunk and not just pushing back with his shoulder. You provide matching resistance for this isometric contraction, being sure that the client is breathing normally throughout.

3. After the isometric push, the stretcher relaxes and breathes in. As he relaxes, he maintains his torso in the starting position.

4. On the exhale, ask him to rotate farther to the right, keeping his head in neutral and his spine lengthened. This increases the stretch of the left trunk rotators.

5. Repeat 2 to 3 times, then reposition the client to do the same stretch for the left trunk rotators.

Trunk Rotators Self-Stretch—Seated

Sit comfortably in a straight back chair. Keeping your spine lengthened and your head in neutral, twist to the right as far as you can, then grab the back of the chair to hold yourself there. Try to twist back to the left, using your trunk, not just your shoulders. After this isometric contraction, twist farther to the right, again using your trunk and not pulling with your arms (figure 6.16).

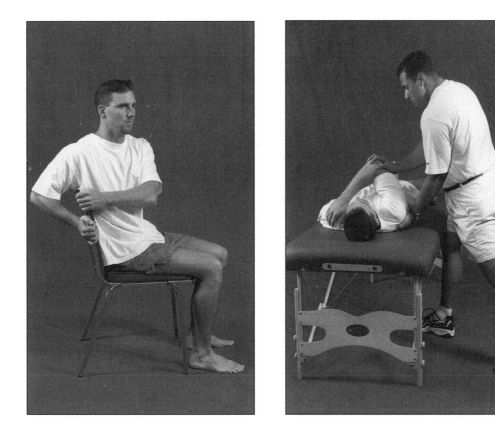

Figure 6.16   Trunk rotators self-stretch.

Figure 6.17   Initiation of the rhomboid stretch, supine.

Rhomboid Stretch—Supine

This stretch is used to improve scapular protraction (movement of the scapula away from the midline).

1. The stretcher is supine. With his right arm flexed at the elbow, he brings his humerus across his chest as far as possible. He may assist this motion by pulling with his left hand. He does not roll his torso up to the left. This lengthens the right rhomboids to their end range.

2. Stand facing his right side. Place your right hand on his right humerus at the elbow. Reach under his back so that your left hand is in firm contact with the body of the right scapula and so that your left fingers grasp its medial border (figure 6.17). Ask the stretcher to begin slowly to try to pull his scapula toward his spine. You provide matching resistance for this isometric contraction, being sure that the client is breathing normally throughout. Be sure he engages his rhomboids and is not just pushing from his arm.

3. After the isometric push, the stretcher relaxes and breathes in. As he relaxes, maintain the scapula and arm in the starting position.

4. On the exhale, ask him to pull his arm farther across his chest, protracting the scapula farther away from the spine and increasing the rhomboid stretch.

5. Repeat 2 to 3 times.

Rhomboid Self-Stretch—Supine or Seated

Flex your arm and shoulder to 90 degrees and bring it across your chest. This pulls your scapula away from your spine and stretches your rhomboids. Use your other hand to hold at your elbow, stabilizing your arm. Try to bring your scapula toward your spine, isometrically contracting your rhomboids. After the isometric contraction, stretch the rhomboids by bringing your arm farther across your chest (figure 6.18).

Quadratus Lumborum (QL) Stretch—Side Lying

The quadratus lumborum has fibers that run vertically and in two diagonals. This stretch is primarily for the vertical fibers, which make up the bulk of the muscle. It works best if the hip abductors are stretched first (see pages 63-64).

1. The stretcher is lying on his left side, with his back at the edge of the table and his right leg hyperextended and hanging over the edge of the table. Be sure he keeps his hips stacked vertically on top of each other. He reaches his right arm up over his head. This lengthens the right QL.

If the stretcher experiences any low back pain in this position, he may bend forward from the waist to round his low back while keeping his leg hanging off the edge of the table.

2. Stand behind the stretcher to keep him from falling off the table! Cross your arms and place your left hand against his right iliac crest; your right hand is spread wide and placed on the lateral aspect of his rib cage (figure 6.19).

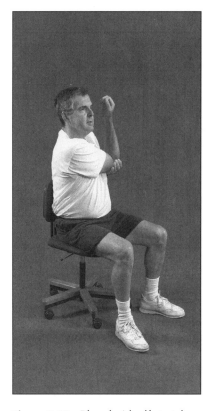

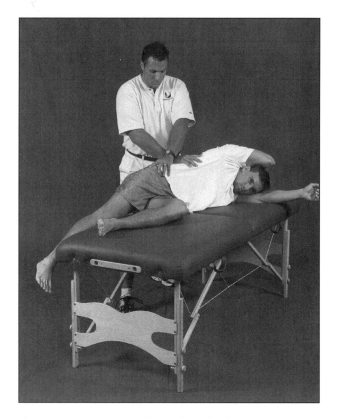

Figure 6.18 Rhomboid self-stretch.

Figure 6.19 Initiation of the quadratus lumborum stretch, side lying.

3. Stretcher education begins now. Your goal is to have him contract the right QL by bringing the hip and the ribs toward each other. He is side bending and "hiking" his hip at the same time. Many people have difficulty doing this, so you may need to break the motion into separate components and work with him until he can do each motion separately, then combine them. Be patient and creative.

4. Once the stretcher can perform the motion, ask him to begin slowly to try to bring the top of his hip and his rib cage toward each other. You apply matching resistance to prevent any motion from occurring. You control the force of the push.

5. After the isometric push, the stretcher relaxes and inhales deeply. As he relaxes, allow his leg (and his hip) to drop toward the floor.

6. On the exhale, ask the client to pull his foot closer to the floor and reach farther up over his head to increase the stretch on the right QL.

7. Repeat 2 to 3 times.

Quadratus Lumborum Self-Stretch—Seated

Sit comfortably, with your spine lengthened. Place a towel or strap under your left foot, and hold the other end in your left hand. Side bend to the left as far as you can, taking up any slack in the strap (figure 6.20). This lengthens the right QL. Using the strap to prevent your motion, try to bend up to the right, isometrically contracting the right QL. Deepen the stretch by bending farther to the left.

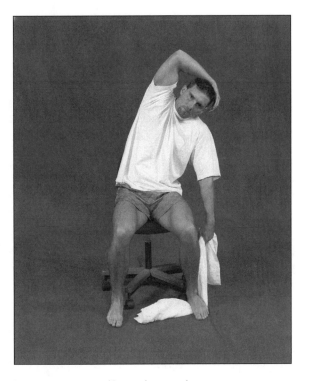

Figure 6.20   QL self-stretch, seated.

Latissimus Dorsi Stretch—Prone

This stretch mimics the "lat pull-down" used to strengthen the lats and is used to increase range of motion in flexion and external rotation of the humerus.

1. The stretcher is prone on the table, with his arms outstretched (in the "diving" position) and externally rotated. This position lengthens the lats to their end range.

2. Using a stable front-to-back stance, grasp the stretcher's arms or wrists securely (figure 6.21). Direct the stretcher to begin slowly to try and pull his arms toward his feet and rotate them internally, engaging the lats bilaterally.

3. After the isometric pull, the stretcher relaxes and breathes in.

4. On the exhale, ask the stretcher to reach farther forward (away from his feet) and rotate his arms more laterally, deepening the stretch of the latissimus dorsi.

5. Repeat 2 to 3 times.

Latissimus Dorsi Stretch—Side Lying

1. The stretcher is side lying on his left side, with his right arm abducted and behind his head, elbow bent. His shoulders and hips are stacked vertically, his low back is flat, and his knees are bent for comfort and stability. This position lengthens the latissimus to its end range.

2. Stand behind the stretcher and grasp his elbow with your left hand. Place your right hand at his hip (figure 6.22). Ask the stretcher to try to push his right arm toward the

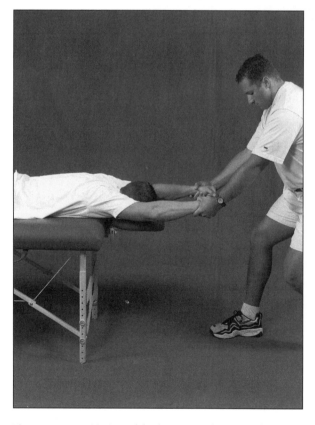

Figure 6.21 Initiation of the latissimus dorsi stretch, prone.

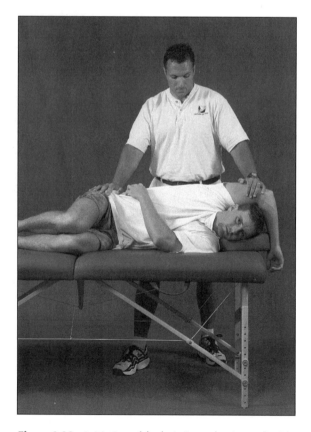

Figure 6.22 Initiation of the latissimus dorsi stretch, side lying.

ceiling. You provide matching resistance for this isometric contraction, being sure that the stretcher is breathing normally throughout.

3. After the isometric push, the stretcher relaxes and breathes in. As he relaxes, the arm may drop toward the floor or be maintained in the starting position.

4. On the exhale, ask the stretcher to reach farther toward the floor, deepening the stretch of the latissimus dorsi.

5. Repeat 2 to 3 times.

Latissimus Dorsi Self-Stretch—Seated

This stretch may be done seated or standing, but the seated position stabilizes your hips to help your biomechanics. Keep your back and neck lengthened and bring your right arm, elbow bent, up behind your head, trying to reach your left shoulder. Grab your right elbow with your left hand (figure 6.23). Attempt to bring your right arm down to your right side, resisting with your left hand. Following the isometric contraction, reach your right arm farther to the left to increase the stretch on the right latissimus dorsi.

To increase the stretch even more, side bend to the left.

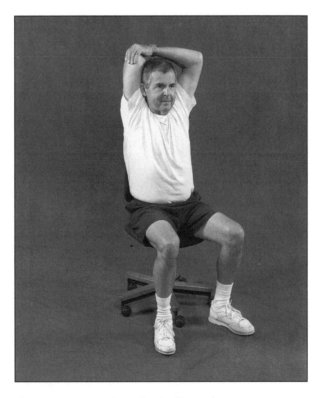

Figure 6.23 Latissimus dorsi self-stretch.

THORACIC AND LUMBAR AREA

Chapter 7

PNF in Physical Therapy

Rehabilitation involves much more than simply regaining range of motion. It must also work on strength, speed, endurance, and normal function. As used in physical therapy, PNF works with the central and peripheral nervous systems, spinal reflex mechanisms, cortical stimulation, integration of the proprioceptive system, and the musculoskeletal system, to name only a few. A key difference between PNF and other methods of strengthening and stretching is that PNF incorporates spiral and diagonal patterns of motion, which are much more functional.

The role of PNF in rehabilitation and in physical therapy is quite broad. A physical therapist may use PNF techniques to treat a newborn with a congenital neurological dysfunction, a 90-year-old stroke victim, a 21-year-old motorcycle accident victim with a severe closed head injury, or a 42-year-old who has had surgery for a brain tumor. PNF stretching is just one aspect of PNF and includes several passive, active, and active-assisted methods to stretch soft tissues.

The primary focus of this book is on a "healthy" population. The facilitated stretching that has been presented in previous chapters is one PNF technique of the many that are used by skilled practitioners. The purpose of this chapter is to present an overview of the many ways that PNF techniques are used in the rehabilitation process. You'll see that PNF is a multilayered modality that is useful in every stage of rehabilitation.

Although this chapter can't give you a complete working knowledge of PNF as it is employed during rehabilitation, you'll receive an informative overview.

In this chapter we'll

- discuss the goal of rehabilitation,

- provide examples of the variety of conditions that benefit from PNF,

- discuss modalities used in rehabilitating sports injuries, and

- examine specific rehabilitation scenarios to provide an in-depth look at the way a program is developed to restore pain-free motion, flexibility, strength, endurance, and speed.

Goal of Rehabilitation

The goal of a rehabilitation program is to restore the injured person to preinjury status or better. Results are charted through preinjury and postinjury comparisons of pain level, strength, range of motion, and function. These criteria are monitored closely to ensure that the patient is progressing toward preinjury status. The initial rehabilitation program will be altered as necessary during treatment to keep the patient on track in the healing process.

During rehabilitation, a full range of PNF techniques may be used to stretch and strengthen muscles in a functional, coordinated manner. Some of the specific PNF techniques include approximation, traction, hold-relax active motion, rhythmic initiation, rhythmic stabilization, rhythmic rotation, slow reversal, slow reversal hold, quick reversal, contract-relax, and hold-relax. (For further information about these techniques, consult Voss et al. 1985.)

Flexibility is an important component of the physiological function of muscle. Although very little scientific data are available to prove that good flexibility prevents injuries, most practitioners agree that it does. From a physics standpoint, a strong, long muscle will produce more total work than a strong, short muscle.

The biomechanics and the dynamics of sports are too complex to allow us to simplify our rehabilitation programs down to only strength and flexibility. We must also address psychomotor function, agility, proprioception, power, endurance, coordination, specific joint mechanics, and core stability, among many variables, when rehabilitating an injured person. Sport-specific training is used toward the end stages of rehabilitation to better prepare an athlete for practice and, ultimately, competition. Work-specific training (work hardening) is used in a similar fashion for the injured worker, with the ultimate goal being to return him to full duties at work.

Using PNF With Many Conditions

Although physical therapy uses conventional passive and active stretching as part of a total rehabilitation program, PNF stretching and strengthening techniques are far more common. PNF techniques allow more "hands-on" training, which gives the therapist a more accurate "feel" of how the tissues and joints are moving, compensating, or both. The therapist can better isolate specific tissues to treat in a more efficient manner using PNF techniques.

Physical therapy has evolved in recent years away from "symptom-driven" treatment such as ultrasound, electrical stimulation, heat, and cold. Rather, we assess and treat function from both a practical standpoint and a biomechanical perspective. This involves assessment of both soft tissues and joints.

Many conditions lend themselves to PNF techniques. For example, a person who sustains a severe head injury or a stroke resulting in central nervous system damage (to the brain or spinal cord) will require extensive rehabilitation to retrain damaged neuromuscular pathways. PNF is perhaps the most valuable tool for restoring normal movement patterns, strength, endurance, and, ultimately, full function.

Rehabilitation of a back injury requires segmental and multisegmental stabilization techniques, which are found in the PNF repertoire. After immobilization of a fracture, we need to restore full range of motion, strength, and function in that segment of the body affected either directly or indirectly. PNF can be invaluable in achieving these goals. A baseball pitcher with a torn rotator cuff will require aggressive PNF strengthening and stretching after surgery to be able to return to throwing. A therapist can use PNF stretching to help a burn patient improve joint ROM by mobilizing scars and stretching skin grafts. These examples illustrate but a few of the ways PNF can be incorporated into a rehabilitation program.

The Rehabilitation Process

Now that you have a better appreciation for the role PNF plays in rehabilitation, we'll discuss the general guidelines for rehabilitating an overuse sports injury. Whatever your sport—tennis, running, biking, swimming, hiking, etc.—you've probably experienced pain because of overuse—that is, "too much, too soon." Whenever you increase the intensity or the duration of exercise, you run the risk of soft tissue injury, which results in inflammation.

Control Inflammation

Inflammation is your body's normal response to injury, but it must be controlled. Histamine released into the injured area causes blood vessels to dilate, bringing more nutrients to the injury site to help heal the tissues but also causing swelling. Pain then results from pressure on the free nerve endings in the swollen area. (*Note:* Swelling can also be the result of bleeding from larger vessels or trauma to ligaments or bone. Our discussion is focused on microvascular damage caused by minor overuse injuries.) Swelling also interferes with healing by reducing the oxygen supply to the injured tissue. Minor overuse injuries usually heal by themselves with proper rest and perhaps the use of ice and nonsteroidal anti-inflammatory medication. Problems arise when we ignore these mild symptoms and continue to train or perform the activity that caused the initial response.

A physical therapist or certified athletic trainer usually sees patients with inflammation after they've seen a doctor for pain or injury that "just won't go away" or that is getting worse. The initial goals in therapy are to reduce the inflammation (which will reduce the pain) and concomitantly restore passive range of motion.

There are a number of ways to reduce inflammation. Cold is the most widely used modality to control inflammation and swelling, reduce muscle spasm, and relieve pain. It's typically applied using ice packs or ice massage.

Several electrical modalities can be helpful, such as electrical stimulation (AC-alternating current—low frequency, high frequency, surged, and varying wave forms), iontophoresis (delivery of medication via direct current), phonophoresis (delivery of medication via ultrasound), MENS (microcurrent), and many more "magic boxes" of all shapes and sizes.

Gentle, passive ROM exercise helps reduce joint pain and swelling. Isometric exercise helps pump away by-products and metabolites via the one-way valve system in the venous and lymphatic systems.

Address Scar Tissue Formation

Once inflammation is reduced, scar tissue formation, weakness, and joint restrictions must be addressed. Scar tissue forms to replace normal tissue that has been injured. Scar formation is minimized when the area is rested appropriately, but once it's formed, we must make the best of it. Normal collagen (tendons and ligaments are made of this) is a very tight, organized matrix with tremendous tensile strength. Scar tissue, on the other hand, is composed of a disorganized, random array of collagen, with a weaker tensile property. If the injury is not treated properly and promptly, this weaker tensile property contributes to reinjury. Deep transverse friction massage can be employed to move and stretch this scar tissue to make it more functional.

Evaluate Joint Mechanics

Next, joint mechanics, namely osteokinematics (ROM) and arthrokinematics (sliding, gliding, and rolling of joint surfaces) are evaluated and restored if restrictions are present.

Use Heat

When acute inflammation has subsided, heat (deep or superficial) is often used to enhance blood flow to the area, resulting in increased elastic properties of the soft tissues for more effective stretching. Ultrasound and diathermy are deep forms of heat. Moist heat packs, warm whirlpools, and paraffin wax are used for more superficial forms of heat. Once the tissue has been heated, PNF techniques can be used to effectively lengthen it without pain. This accomplishes two goals of rehabilitation: to reduce pain and restore normal ROM.

Strengthen Muscles

Once we achieve full joint mobility and soft tissue flexibility (length), our focus shifts toward muscle strengthening. A strengthening program may include the use of isokinetic devices, weight machines, sport cords (surgical tubing is quite versatile), and free weights. PNF is perhaps the most efficient means of achieving strength gains in a specific area.

Most of the "machines" available fail to address one of the most important components of strengthening—the rotational movements of a functional pattern. These machines, for the most part, only strengthen major muscle groups in one or two planes of motion. The machines do not stress the stabilization of proximal (close to the torso) structures that are crucial for proper function and maximal efficiency of the extremities. Several PNF techniques promote proximal stabilization (rhythmic stabilization and approximation, for example), whereas machines actually eliminate this important action when the person is strapped to the machine and the straps do all this work.

A Typical PNF Rehabilitation Session

Although each injured athlete has specific needs that must be met during a rehabilitation program, certain commonalities exist in every case. Certain modalities are used in a particular phase of rehabilitation, and some are used throughout a treatment program. The following discussion is by no means a thorough look at the possible treatment programs that might be designed for the same injury. It is only an outline of a program.

• *Warm-up.* Once the acute inflammation of an injury has subsided, a typical session may begin by warming the joint and muscles by applying a moist heat pack for 20 minutes, an ultrasound for 5 to 10 minutes, or some light exercise for 10 minutes, using pulleys, the upper body ergometer (UBE), or the stationary bike.

• *Preliminary mobilization.* Once the area is sufficiently warmed up, we can begin stretching. When treating a shoulder injury, we prefer to first have the patient use a T-bar (PVC tubing shaped as a T) with an independent self-stretching routine. Next, we employ joint mobilization techniques to improve joint arthrokinematics so that PNF stretching will be more effective and comfortable. Once the muscles have adequate blood profusion (are warmed up) and the joint is mobile, we are ready to begin PNF stretching and strengthening.

• *PNF stretching and strengthening.* We prefer to alternate sets of PNF stretching and strengthening. Depending on the athlete's fitness level and what we are trying to emphasize (strength, power, endurance), we may complete several sets of 10, 20, 30, or more repetitions on several patterns. Which patterns we use depend on our assessment as to which muscles are weaker, tighter, and so on.

• *Cryotherapy.* Most clinicians prefer to ice the injured area after the session in case of inflammation caused by the rehabilitation program. Ice can be applied using ice massage directly to the area for 5 to 10 minutes or an ice bag for no more than 20 to 30 minutes.

• *General conditioning.* We also include general strengthening and cardiovascular conditioning of the entire body in the rehabilitation program. Generally, people are deconditioned after an injury because they've been unable to participate in their sport. The body will heal faster if it's in good general condition. Cardiovascular conditioning is usually done using a stationary bicycle, stair climber, treadmill, UBE, or swimming pool. A general weight training program is used for building or maintaining strength, keeping in mind any restrictions related to the injured area.

• *Sport-specific training.* Finally, once a functional strength base is achieved and the patient has full range of motion without pain, we progress to the activity itself, using sport-specific training. We're now ready, for example, to initiate an interval throwing program for a baseball pitcher or throwing a football (this slows down the throwing motion velocity). A runner, cyclist, or tennis player would use a similar progressive interval program to gradually return to full activity. A maintenance program is necessary to prevent a reoccurrence of the injury and can usually be effective when done three times per week in conjunction with a normal training program.

Rehabilitating a Pitcher: PNF in Practice

As an example, let's take a baseball pitcher following arthroscopic decompression of the subacromial joint, a common procedure with rotator cuff injuries. Putting this athlete on a machine to build muscle strength will do very little for the scapulothoracic musculature. Free weights and machines can work the muscles in only one or two planes of motion, but the pitching motion occurs in a three-dimensional plane. There are many ways in which PNF allows us to build strength, endurance, and power in a functional three-dimensional manner.

Muscles Used in Pitching

The primary muscles responsible for accelerating the arm during pitching are the pectoralis major, latissimus dorsi, teres major, subscapularis, and triceps brachii. D1 and D2 extension patterns will incorporate all but one of these, the triceps brachii. The triceps only work isometrically when we carry out the motion with the elbow extended. A nice feature of PNF is that we can modify the techniques to include all the muscles that need work. Therefore, we can start either D1 or D2 extension with the elbow flexed to strengthen the triceps concentrically.

The other major action of the pitching motion is deceleration after the ball is released. The primary muscles responsible for this action are the biceps brachii, deltoid, supraspinatus, infraspinatus, teres minor, and the scapular stabilizers (which we will discuss later). The biceps decelerates the elbow and the glenohumeral joint. The supraspinatus, infraspinatus, and teres minor, in addition to dynamically stabilizing the glenohumeral joint during the cocking and acceleration phase, also decelerate the glenohumeral joint after release of the ball. Therefore, it is extremely important to strengthen these muscles, commonly referred to as the rotator cuff, both concentrically and eccentrically. We do this by supplementing the PNF strengthening regimen with resistive exercises (e.g. free weights, surgical tubing) to build eccentric as well as concentric strength.

When rehabilitating the throwing shoulder, we must also be aware of the importance of the scapular stabilizing muscles. The primary stabilizers (figure 7.1) are the rhomboids, trapezius, levator scapula, and serratus anterior. From an anatomical and musculoskeletal standpoint, the arm is fairly useless without a strong base of support, which the scapula provides. If the muscles surrounding the

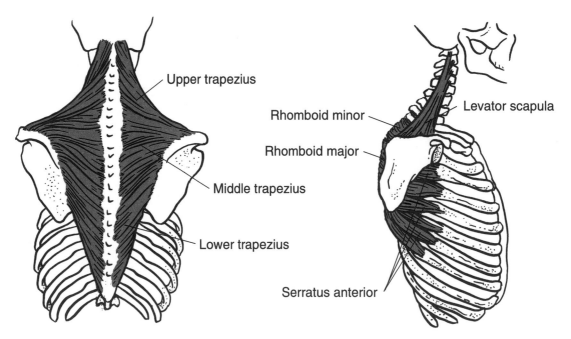

Figure 7.1   Scapular stabilizers: trapezius, rhomboids, levator scapula, and serratus anterior.

scapula are weak, the muscles of the shoulder joint cannot work efficiently. The shoulder muscles are not only at a biomechanical disadvantage with weak scapular muscles, but they may also be at higher risk of injury or reinjury. Therefore, it is imperative to include the scapular muscles during rehabilitation.

Using PNF to Rehabilitate a Pitcher

By using the D2 extension pattern (figure 7.2a), we can simulate the motion a pitcher uses while delivering a screwball (figure 7.2b). By reversing the rotation

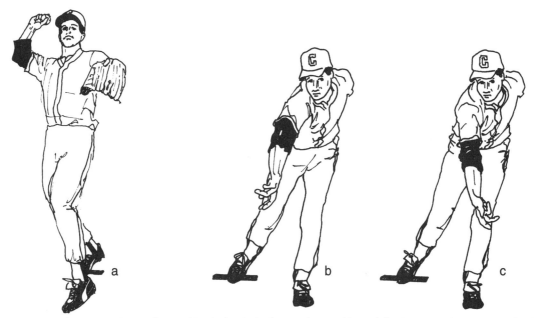

Figure 7.2   (a) When preparing to throw, this pitcher is in the starting position of the D2 extension pattern. (b) Pitching a screwball uses the normal D2 extension. (c) Pitching a curveball reverses the usual rotation of D2 extension.

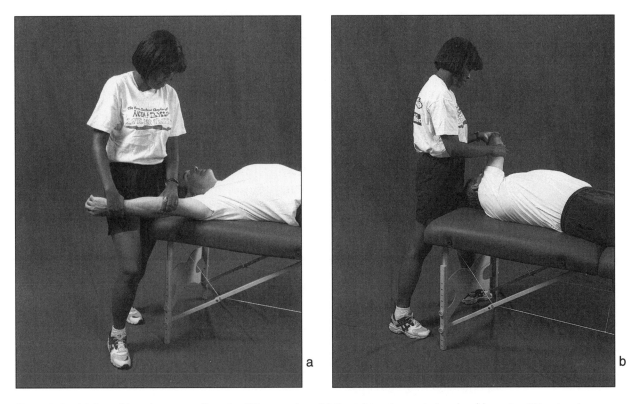

Figure 7.3 (a) Stretching the pectoralis using D2 extension. (b) Stretching the posterior shoulder using D1 extension.

component of D2 extension, we can simulate a curveball (figure 7.2c). By resisting either D1 or D2 flexion patterns eccentrically, we are building the deceleration muscles, which are critical following release of the ball.

We can instruct the pitcher in several prone, sitting, or standing exercises that emphasize adduction of the scapula and horizontal abduction of the shoulder using free weights, surgical tubing, or even some machines. Early in the rehabilitation program, we can initiate scapular stabilization using rhythmic stabilization, rhythmic initiation, and approximation of the shoulder joint. All these PNF techniques can achieve the desired outcome under the hands of a trained clinician.

Frequently, athletes who throw a great deal have strong, tight anterior (accelerating) muscles and relatively weak posterior muscles, creating significant muscle imbalance. PNF stretching can play an important role in correcting this imbalance. For example, to gain maximal elongation of the pectoralis major, we use facilitated stretching at the beginning of D2 extension (figure 7.3a). If the posterior glenohumeral joint capsule is tight, we use facilitated stretching at the beginning position of D1 extension (figure 7.3b).

Rehabilitating a Runner: PNF in Practice

Patellofemoral pain (pain in and around the knee) is probably the most common complaint involving the knee. There are usually multiple contributing factors, including lack of flexibility. Many of these contributing factors will be presented here along with treatment remedies.

Examination

The first thing we (physical therapists) do is evaluate the patient to determine the cause of the problem. Invariably some type of inflammatory process is causing the pain. This inflammation can be a result of many things, but training errors are the most common cause of knee pain.

The subjective examination includes any information that the patient can give us. We try our best to isolate the cause of pain by asking the patient about the onset (acute or chronic), the quality and intensity of the pain/symptoms, and what activities make it better or worse.

Next, an objective physical examination is done that includes assessment of the musculoskeletal system. Also, diagnostic testing results are reviewed, such as X rays that could show advanced degenerative changes in the joints. Then we put all the pieces together and make an overall assessment of the condition. Finally, we devise a treatment plan based on our assessment.

Case Presentation

In this case, a 28-year-old, national-class female distance runner comes in with complaints of right knee pain during the past two to three weeks. It started over the course of two days and has gotten to the point where she can no longer run hills or continue her interval training. It's worse in the morning and after she has been sitting too long at work. She added interval training to her training program two weeks ago. She has also been running hills to improve her aerobic power. She has never done interval training before this time.

Orthotics were fitted by a podiatrist two years ago because of tendinitis in her ankle. She also has a history of some low back pain and iliotibial (IT) band tendinitis, all involving the right side.

Findings

Examination of the patient shows her to walk with a slight limp on the right side. She experiences pain when she tries to squat down and bend her right knee, although she has full knee range of motion. Flexibility testing reveals tightness in her calf, hamstrings, tensor fascia latae/iliotibial band, and hip external rotators.

She has weakness in the hip extensors and internal rotators. Her VMO (vastus medialis oblique) is atrophied, with poor definition. Poor control is apparent while lowering herself into a partially squatted position on the right leg. Functional weakness is noted in the posterior tibialis. Examination of the right foot reveals excessive pronation, with restriction of the subtalar joint. Observation of her running on the treadmill shows a severe compensation on the right side after 15 minutes. Her right foot rotated outward, and she could not bend the right knee as much during swing-through phase.

Palpation reveals marked tenderness in the following areas, all on the right side: lateral patellofemoral joint, iliotibial band, vastus lateralis, posterior tibialis tendon, and the iliopsoas. Biomechanical testing of the patellofemoral joint shows an increased Q-angle on the right side, which contributes to excessive lateral tracking of the patella. The patella is also laterally tilted and externally rotated when in the neutral position. Closer inspection of the patella shows weakness in the articularis genus muscle because of an impingement of the synovium at the medial retinaculum. Adverse neural tension testing (Butler 1991; Elvey 1986) of the sciatic nerve reveals restriction of the neural tissues in the right leg by 50 percent.

Treatment

The first issue to be addressed is the inflammation itself. Her doctor has prescribed a nonsteroidal anti-inflammatory medication, which she just started taking. We initiate treatment to help reduce inflammation, including electrical stimulation, ice, and iontophoresis.

Concomitantly, the flexibility deficiencies are addressed. A home program is started immediately that includes static stretches for the hamstrings, calf, and hip.

Active Rest   As the inflamed tissues are being calmed down, the athlete is asked not to perform the activities that put her over the edge—that is, intervals and hills. An "active rest" program is established to maintain her cardiovascular status as rehabilitation takes place. Cross-training is implemented to include swimming three days per week, biking twice per week, and weight training three days per week.

Strength Training   She comes to the clinic to perform the weight training, which includes specific VMO and hip strengthening exercises, abdominal work, and upper body exercises. The hip extensors, internal rotators, and VMO are all strengthened because they were found to be weak during the initial evaluation. Abdominals are worked because of her previous history of back pain and the poor lower abdominal control (strength) discovered in the evaluation. The upper body is very important in assisting with the running stride, therefore while she is cutting back on actual running, the strength and endurance of her arms are maximized. When she returns to running, this regimen will have prevented further loss of function and perhaps replaced some of the physiological losses that occurred during the rehabilitation period.

PNF Techniques   Each day when she has finished her weight training and cross-training, she is treated in the clinic. Although she is fatigued from the weight lifting, we complete four sets through the full pattern of D1 extension and D2 flexion, which both emphasize internal rotation of the hip. This program counteracts the dominant feature of her running gait: excessive external rotation of the leg.

Flexibility is addressed in the clinic as well. After she does her self-stretches, we use PNF stretching techniques, including contract-relax, hold-relax, and facilitated stretching. The primary muscles worked on are the hamstrings, tensor fascia latae, hip external rotators, and gastrocnemius/soleus. Joint mobilization is performed to the subtalar joint because of the restrictions found there during the evaluation.

Functional Training   The functional weakness of the lower extremity is addressed next. The patient has a "supinatory" weakness, which results in a "pronatory pattern" of the lower extremity. Supination has historically referred only to the foot. In recent years, Gary Gray, PT, (1995) has extended this definition to include a total limb posture of the lower extremity. "Supination" in his work is a "chain reaction" that occurs when the foot hits the ground and includes not only supination of the foot but also external rotation of the hip and knee.

The "supinatory pattern" refers to a functional position of the lower extremity, which includes the pelvis, hip, knee, ankle, and foot. Rarely does supination of the foot and ankle occur without these other movements in the leg. They are all orchestrated together to most efficiently resist the effects of gravity. These movements are interdependent on one another. The functional weakness of her lower extremity is partially addressed during the PNF patterns for the leg; the resistance is focused distally to facilitate the posterior tibialis muscle along with the total leg supinatory motion.

Once a comprehensive functional program is completed addressing the deficiencies she came in with, she is progressed to more and more difficult tasks. This functional progression becomes more and more sport specific to the patient as she approaches the final stages of rehabilitation. In this case, endurance and running activities are stressed.

Patellar Tracking   An additional component in this case is the weakness of the articularis genus muscle, which attaches to the joint capsule of the knee and holds it out of the way as the patella glides superiorly on the femur. Specificity in this case is difficult because the muscle is quite small and is located deep to the quadriceps muscle. Retraining of articularis genus is difficult, but an attempt is made with electrical stimulation and manual input/resistance to the patella to improve tracking. Also, McConnell taping (1986) is employed to improve her kinesthetic awareness of her patellofemoral joint and correct the neutral positional dysfunction noted during the intake evaluation.

Nerve Gliding   Because of the chronic nature of her condition, this patient has also sensitized the sciatic nerve, which is compounding her symptoms. We must restore normal mobility of these tissues for her to completely recover from her injury. This is accomplished by performing nerve gliding exercises to restore full mobility to the sciatic nerve. Nerve gliding is a technique developed by Butler (1991) and Elvey (1986).

Manual Therapy   Finally, the symptomatic psoas muscle on the right is examined, which reveals a lumbopelvic dysfunction caused by compensation patterns. Manual therapy techniques are performed here to correct a pelvic torsion and some lumbar vertebral dysfunction, which has a direct effect on the external rotation problem of the hips.

Rehabilitating a Person With Low Back Pain: PNF in Practice

A large majority of people experience low back pain at some time during their lives. We thought it would be helpful to include this condition in our discussion of PNF and rehabilitation.

Let's take a moderate problem such as a sudden onset of low back pain. A medical doctor may have seen the patient first and prescribed bed rest and nonsteroidal anti-inflammatory drugs (for example, ibuprofen), which is the usual medical treatment. If there was a violent mechanism of injury that could have caused a fracture, X rays would be taken. Or a chiropractor or osteopath may have treated the patient with manipulation techniques. Or the patient may have gone to a massage therapist to relieve the pain.

Examination

Physical therapists first evaluate the patient. No matter the source of the problem, invariably some type of inflammatory process is occurring. We try our best to isolate the cause of pain, which could be from the muscles, fascia, ligaments, disks, nerves, or some combination of these tissues. During our interview with the patient, we ask about the onset (acute or chronic), the quality of the pain, the quantity and magnitude of symptoms, and what activities make the symptoms better or worse.

We then observe how the patient moves, walks, transfers, bends forward, bends backward, and so on. This gives us an idea of his beginning functional level of activity. Once we have an idea of what the pain is like and how it affects his function, we try to isolate the specific structures that are causing the pain. Nerve involvement in the lower back region is often "sciatica," which is inflammation of the sciatic nerve. The patient with this condition usually has varying degrees of pain down the back of the leg. More severe symptoms consist of numbness and weakness in the leg.

We also perform a series of tests to determine any strength loss, sensory changes, muscle spasms, altered soft tissue texture, loss of flexibility, segmental joint restrictions in the lumbar vertebrae, or soft tissue biomechanical abnormalities. These tests are quite involved and take some time, but this is the most thorough method to determine accurately the cause and extent of the injury. Most often, we find joint restrictions creating soft tissue guarding and compensatory movement patterns, all interrelated to one another. Oftentimes if they are not all addressed together, the condition will linger unnecessarily.

Treatment

Once the patient has been evaluated, we proceed to treatment. Initially we may use a combination of ice, electrical stimulation, heat, gentle stretching, and massage to reduce the pain and inflammation. During this early phase, we educate the patient as to the "dos and don'ts" of preventing further aggravation of the injury. We explain what structures are involved and why certain stretches or strengthening exercises are necessary. For example, tight hamstrings are a common factor in low back pain. The hamstrings attach to the pelvis. If they're too tight, they will cause undo strain on the lumbar spine into flexion. This may further aggravate a condition involving the intervertebral disks. Conversely, a tight psoas muscle can lead to increased extension in the lumbar spine because of its attachment on the anterior lumbar vertebrae. Education is paramount in an effective rehabilitation program because once the patient understands why a tight or weak muscle is interfering with his recovery, he will be more likely to carry through with instructions for self-care. A gradual progression of activity is allowed depending on the functional status and the compensatory patterns observed. It may be necessary to strengthen certain areas to function properly without further injury, such as abdominal strengthening to protect the patient's back while lifting or bending.

Once the acute pain subsides, treatment emphasizes restoration of normal movement, both from a specific structural standpoint and from a functional standpoint. We can also begin working more aggressively on restoring both joint and soft tissue movement as well as strength deficiencies related to the problem.

Concomitantly during this phase, we use various manual therapies, soft tissue therapy, and joint mobilization techniques. These can be wide and varied, depending on the practitioner's experience level. For example, it is very common to have the quadratus lumborum, iliopsoas, and piriformis muscles protect and guard the back during the painful, inflammatory phase. Once the initial injury has resolved, these muscles may still be in a "protective mode" and forget to let go. We assist the lengthening and relaxation of these muscles by using facilitated stretching and soft tissue therapy. Some of the deeper muscles are difficult to reach and treat manually. We therefore use facilitated stretching techniques to achieve specific elongation of these muscles and surrounding tissues. Often, this is the only way to achieve the desired effect on these tissues.

Home Program

The patient is next progressed to a home program consisting of

1. gentle self-stretches (bringing the knees to the chest while lying on his back, trunk rotation, and hamstrings, quads, and hip flexor stretches);
2. stabilization exercises (holding the pelvis steady while doing progressively more difficult maneuvers);
3. functional retraining (partial squats while maintaining good posture, sitting against a wall in good posture, lunges with good posture); and
4. strengthening (isometric abdominal bracing, partial crunches, oblique abdominal crunches, leg extensions, and leg curls). During this phase the patient is continually reassessed and progressed to more advanced

exercises as tolerated. Our goal at this point is to continually improve the joint range of motion, flexibility, strength, and ultimately his functional status.

Maintenance

Once normal range of motion, strength, and function is restored, patients are given a comprehensive written maintenance program to assure that they have all the "tools" to minimize the chance of reoccurrence. Our ultimate goal is to never have to treat the injury again. Frequently patients do return with "flare-ups" that may require a specific joint manipulation or soft tissue release, but if they continue with the maintenance program, the severity should be far less than their initial back injury. Their recovery should be much faster because of the improved "resilience" and adaptive potential their musculoskeletal system now possesses. Maintaining an adequate general fitness level (via regular exercise), strength base (home exercises), flexibility (daily home stretches—including facilitated stretching), and posture/lumbar stability (home exercises) will most certainly prove effective.

Summary

As you can see through these cases, which are not that uncommon, there are far too many components of injury and treatment to cover in the context of this chapter. Rather, we hope we have shed some light on the "big picture" and stimulated you to broaden your thinking. There are so many ways to approach musculoskeletal problems; what we have presented is only a slice of them. New, better, and more refined techniques and thought processes are being brought to the forefront all the time. We hope that you explore the use of these techniques, at whatever level is appropriate for your skill and training, and find ways to make them better!

Soft Tissue Therapy and Facilitated Stretching

Injured muscles usually heal by forming scar tissue at the injury site. The final scar is often dense and inflexible and limits pain-free motion. To restore pain-free motion, the scar tissue must be modified in some way. Physicians are generally limited to medication or surgery in their approach to treatment and can do very little about scarring. Many physical therapists still rely on treatments such as ice, heat, ultrasound, and electrical muscle stimulation. These approaches are often effective and many times an important component in the early treatment of soft tissue trauma, but they are inadequate for modifying scar tissue that has formed. Some type of manual therapy, like massage or myofascial release, is necessary to effectively reduce the scar tissue and restore pain-free motion. Facilitated stretching, when used appropriately with manual soft tissue therapy, can increase the likelihood of safely and effectively restoring pain-free motion to muscles that have been injured.

Fibrotic Tissue

Scar tissue or adhesions can develop within and between muscles, fascia, and neural tissues. These adhesions can cause any array of problems from minor periodic discomfort to severe progressive compensatory dysfunction and even nerve damage.

Scar tissue may develop because of acute trauma to the tissues or over time as repetitive stress injury. Although scar tissue formation is a normal response to injury, excessive scarring reduces function and contributes to chronic pain and limitation of movement.

Adhesions are nonfunctional cross-links between fibers within a muscle or between layers of muscle, in fascia, and/or in neural tissues. These cross-links prevent normal motion, and this limitation is often accompanied by pain. Adhesions can form as a result of postural stress, chronic hypertonicity in a muscle, or lack of motion.

Adhesions and scar tissue are terms that are often used interchangeably. We will refer to them collectively as fibrotic tissue in the following discussion.

Release of Fibrotic Tissue

Admittedly, much of what follows is based on clinical experience and anecdotal evidence, not on controlled studies.

Many forms of manual soft tissue therapy are used to reduce the restriction and pain caused by fibrotic tissue. When facilitated stretching is added to the mix, better results can be achieved. This combination of stretching and soft tissue work is used only on chronic injuries and rarely with acute injuries. During the acute phase, we must be careful not to disrupt newly forming scar tissue. Stretching or deep soft tissue work is usually contraindicated until the scar tissue has matured.

A Typical Treatment

A typical treatment scenario for chronic injury would begin with an evaluation of the ROM of the injured area, noting where pain is felt and at what point in the motion it begins. Soft tissue work would then be performed if appropriate. This work is followed by facilitated stretching, within the pain-free range of motion, to attempt to increase the pain-free range. Once the new limits of pain-free motion are achieved using facilitated stretching, a small amount of passive stretch is added to pinpoint the exact area where pain is felt in the stretched tissues. We theorize that this painful area is the site of the fibrotic tissue and may be extremely small. Once this area is located, the passive stretch is released slightly until the patient is once again at the pain-free end of range. Specific soft tissue techniques to release the fibrosis (such as transverse friction massage) can then be used on the exact site of the pain. This treatment is immediately followed by gentle active or passive movement to lengthen the treated tissue to a new pain-free range. Another round of facilitated stretching is then initiated. In most cases, the pain-free range of motion will increase again as a result of this combination of techniques.

Releasing the Scalenes

A specific example may be helpful here. Remember, this treatment is used only with chronic injuries, not acute ones. You're treating a patient with chronic pain and limited cervical range of motion secondary to whiplash injuries sustained in an auto accident; specifically, when she laterally flexes to the left, she feels pain on the right side of her neck. She has been medically evaluated, and structural problems, such as a vertebral or disk-related cause for the pain, have been ruled out. This pain pattern, then, would indicate that pain is the result of injured soft tissues, probably the right scalenes. Treatment begins with general soft tissue work to release tension and warm up the muscles of the neck. Then, with the patient supine on the treatment table, you ask her to laterally flex to the left as far as she can without pain. Use facilitated stretching for the right scalenes to try to increase her pain-free range in lateral flexion to the left (see the scalene stretch, page 100).

Following this stretch, whether or not you've gained more range of motion, you laterally flex her to the left passively, just far enough for her to pinpoint the painful area that now limits her motion. Once located, release the passive stretch slightly so that she is once again in a position of comfort. Now you apply friction massage, or a similar technique, to release the fibrotic tissue causing the pain and limitation. After this treatment, ask the client to actively move farther into pain-free lateral flexion to the left, or gently move her passively. She should be able to increase her pain-free range following this soft tissue treatment, but not always. At whatever her pain-free range now is, initiate another round of facilitated stretching to further increase her pain-free range of motion.

Releasing the Hamstrings

Another example of this treatment would involve a client with a chronic hamstring pull, possibly caused by a training error that resulted in an inflammatory response and subsequent fibrotic tissue formation in the belly of the hamstrings. Examination reveals less flexibility in the hamstring with pain associated from the fibrotic adhesions.

Typical treatment may consist of soft tissue work to the hamstrings, heat or ice, and self-directed stretching at home. If he does not respond to this scenario, you can add facilitated stretching immediately following your soft tissue work.

In the supine position, have him actively flex his hip with the knee extended to the point where he feels the restriction. Perform several sets of facilitated stretching on the involved hamstring.

If you want to emphasize the medial hamstring more, use the spiral pattern for D2 extension (see page 70), which will focus the isometric effort and the subsequent stretch to the medial hamstring. To emphasize the lateral hamstrings, use D1 extension. The exact position of the leg in these patterns can be fine-tuned to work directly through the line of restriction felt by the client.

Once you've completed the stretching, you can once again employ specific soft tissue work to continue to release adhesions in the hamstrings. Stretch the hamstrings passively just to the point of pain or restriction so that the client can identify the exact site. Release the passive stretch slightly so that the client is once again in a position of comfort, and begin your specific soft tissue work. Once completed, try once again to increase the pain-free range of motion, using facilitated stretching.

Summary

This combination of facilitated stretching and soft tissue therapy reduces fibrotic tissue more completely than either technique alone. Soft tissue therapies, such as deep transverse friction, have long been used to break down excessive scar tissue or to free adhesions from surrounding tissues and/or bone. We hypothesize that the soft tissue work breaks free some of the fibrosis and that additional cross-links are released with the application of facilitated stretching immediately following. In a sense, the soft tissue work softens up the fibrotic tissue so that stretching is capable of "snapping" fibers that have not been released through the manual technique.

Reviewing the Literature

PNF was developed through trial and error, in a clinical setting, based on hypotheses formed by Dr. Herman Kabat from his synthesis of "the work of (Arnold) Gesell and (George) Coghill on motor development, the findings of (Charles) Sherrington and (Ivan) Pavlov on habit action and reflexes, and the work of (Ernst) Gellhorn on proprioception and cortically controlled movement" (Surburg 1981, 115-16). The technique evolved during the 1950s to include only those patterns of movement that worked most effectively with patients. The patterns, by no coincidence, are similar to the functional patterns that occur naturally in daily activities. It was only after PNF was in wide use that controlled studies were undertaken to examine its effectiveness and to see whether the neurophysiological principles on which it was based could be validated.

In this appendix, we will

- examine arguments against PNF stretching,
- examine evidence supporting PNF stretching, and
- consider the efficacy of PNF stretching today.

Current Research

In recent years, researchers have begun to study PNF stretching in more detail to see whether it actually is more effective than other types of stretching and, if it is more effective, to determine the role of the neurological mechanisms proposed by Kabat.

As research commonly does, many of these studies raise more questions than they answer. But controversy and unanswered questions are beneficial because they stimulate thought, discussion, and further investigation of the mechanisms at work.

Arguments Against PNF Stretching

A number of studies have investigated whether PNF stretching is more effective than other types of stretching. None of the studies I reviewed found PNF to be less effective than other types. However, several researchers recommend other types of stretching over PNF for two reasons:

- PNF stretching is no more effective than other forms of stretching and is too complex.
- There are risks of injury that other forms of stretching eliminate.

PNF Stretching Is Too Complex

The following studies have concluded that, although PNF works, it is no more effective than other types of stretching. Many of these authors believe that, because PNF is more complicated to use, it's better to use the more conventional forms of stretching.

Medeiros, Smidt, Burmeister, and Soderberg (1977) compared the effects of passive stretching versus isometric contractions on range of motion at the hip joint. The testing indicated that both groups significantly increased hip flexion compared with the control group, but there was no significant difference in the gains made by the isometric group compared with the passive stretch group.

In 1984, Lucas and Koslow conducted a study comparing static, dynamic, and PNF stretching. They found that all three types of stretching were effective in increasing the flexibility of the hamstrings and gastrocnemius muscles and that no method produced significantly superior results. They also noted that total stretching time may be a factor in the effectiveness of a particular method. They referred to two studies with short treatment times (18 and 12 minutes) that found PNF to be better, compared with their own study and one other with longer treatment times (105 and 90 minutes) that found no significant differences among the three types of stretching. Condon and Hutton (1987) compared static stretching and three PNF techniques for increasing dorsiflexion of the ankle and concluded that there was no significant difference among techniques.

PNF Stretching Is Too Risky

Several authors have discussed possible risks inherent in using PNF techniques. Their concerns are important and must be considered if we are to avoid injury when using PNF stretching.

Increased EMG Activity   Beaulieu (1981) points out that the isometric contraction preceding a PNF stretch has been shown by Moore and Hutton (1980) to promote higher electromyographic (EMG) readings in the target muscle and, theoretically, puts the muscle more at risk of injury during the stretch phase. (Electromyography is a way of measuring the electrical activity of a muscle. A relaxed muscle is quieter electrically than an active one.)

Investigators in two other EMG studies (Condon and Hutton 1987; Osternig, Robertson, Troxel, and Hansen 1987) also noted higher EMG readings in the target muscle during the antagonist contraction that lengthens the target muscle. These findings seem to indicate that the target muscle is less relaxed following an isometric contraction, that reciprocal inhibition is not occurring as the antagonist contracts, or both. Accordingly, these authors all recommend static stretching as being safer than PNF stretching.

Inattentive Partners   Surburg (1983) discusses the potential injury risks associated with partner (passive) stretching. He believes that lack of attention, improper training, and faulty performance of the techniques are the major factors that contribute to the risk of injury when athletes help one another stretch. He correctly points out that these considerations apply to any stretching technique.

Cardiovascular Complications   Cornelius (1983) mentions the potential risk of increased systolic blood pressure as a result of the valsalva phenomenon during the isometric contraction phase of PNF stretching and the implications raised for those suffering from hypertension. (The valsalva phenomenon occurs when you try to exhale against a closed glottis, as often happens when performing an isometric contraction or lifting a heavy weight. This sets up a series of reactions that can lead to a momentary increase in blood pressure.) However, in a later study (Cornelius and Craft-Hamm 1988) he determined that increases in blood pressure were not significant compared with baseline measures and that the short duration of PNF stretching techniques produced no risks for people who have hypertension without other symptoms.

Cornelius, Jensen, and Odell (1995) monitored systolic and diastolic blood pressure in nonhypertensive subjects performing a variety of PNF hamstring stretches. They found that two rounds of stretching had no effect on blood pressure but that a third round increased systolic pressure.

Neurological Studies

Research has also been done to determine whether the neurological mechanisms thought to be responsible for the effectiveness of PNF techniques are, in fact, responsible. The studies we reviewed throw into question the basic assumptions upon which PNF techniques are based.

Sapega, Quedenfeld, Moyer, and Butler (1981) reviewed relevant research on the factors that contribute to range of motion. They state that "the weight of laboratory evidence indicates that when a relaxed muscle is physically stretched, most, if not all, of the resistance to stretch is derived from the extensive connective tissue framework and sheathing within and around the muscle, not from the myofibrillar elements" (58).

Taylor, Dalton, Seaber, and Garrett (1990) conducted a creative study of the viscoelastic properties of muscle-tendon units and how they are affected by stretching. These authors believe that the viscoelastic properties of the muscle-tendon unit are responsible for the gains made through stretching. Their results indicate that reflex activity has no influence on the results of several stretching procedures.

A series of studies by various researchers using electromyography found levels of electrical activity in the target muscle that indicate the absence of reciprocal or autogenic inhibition during PNF procedures (Moore and Hutton 1980; Cornelius 1983; Condon and Hutton 1987; Osternig et al. 1987 and 1990).

These neurological studies raise serious questions about the validity of Kabat's and others' hypotheses concerning mechanisms like the stretch reflex, reciprocal innervation, and autogenic inhibition and their contribution to the effectiveness of PNF techniques.

Evidence Supporting PNF Stretching

Eight of the fourteen studies we reviewed (57 percent) found that PNF stretching is significantly more effective for increasing ROM and flexibility than static, ballistic, or passive stretching. For example, Tanigawa (1972) compared passive stretching with PNF stretching for the hamstrings. He determined that PNF stretching increased passive hip flexion faster and to a greater extent than did passive stretching.

Moore and Hutton (1980) investigated the differences between static stretching and two PNF stretching techniques using electromyography. Although their findings raised questions about the value of using isometric contraction prior to a stretch, their results indicated that CRAC stretches were more effective than static stretching for improving flexibility.

In 1982, Sady, Wortman, and Blanke reported their study comparing ballistic, static, and PNF stretching on the flexibility of the shoulder, trunk, and hamstring muscles. They found that only the PNF technique (CRAC) significantly increased range of motion compared with the control group. These researchers also noted that individual flexibility changed from day to day, compared with the baseline flexibility established for each subject in the study. In addition, they found flexibility to be highly variable within the body. Their subjects increased flexibility in the hamstrings to a greater extent than in the trunk muscles. They theorized that this may be due to daily postural mechanics that demand more flexibility of the trunk muscles than the hamstrings. Therefore, the hamstrings have a greater range of improvement possible.

Prentice (1983) compared static stretching and PNF stretching for increasing flexibility at the hip joint and found that while both methods were effective, PNF was significantly better than static stretching. Cornelius and Craft-Hamm (1988) compared passive stretching and three types of PNF stretching while investigating their effects on arterial blood pressure. They determined that the PNF techniques were more effective than passive stretching. They also found that there were no significant increases in arterial blood pressure during PNF and concluded that the benefits of PNF stretching outweigh any potential risk of elevated blood pressure.

A study done by Etnyre and Abraham (1986a) compared static stretching to PNF stretching (CR and CRAC) for increasing ROM at the ankle joint. They determined that CRAC is more effective than CR, which is more effective than static stretching, for improving dorsiflexion at the ankle. In another study by Etnyre and Abraham (1986b), they compared the effects of static stretching and two types of PNF stretching on the Hoffmann reflex (H-reflex), "with the objective of revealing central nervous system influences promoting muscle compliance to lengthening." They again concluded that CRAC techniques "provide the greatest potential for muscle lengthening." In two similar EMG studies (1987, 1990), Osternig, Robertson, Troxel, and Hansen concluded that PNF stretching is more effective than static stretching, although PNF evokes higher EMG activity in the target muscle.

Efficacy of PNF Today

If the conflicting reports of all these investigators are confusing, don't worry. It's common in research of this type that some studies are positive and others negative. Even though we may not fully understand how or why PNF techniques work, it is clear that, at the minimum, PNF stretching is as effective as other types of stretching. We also need to recognize that research often lags behind practical experience. Many therapists who use PNF stretching believe strongly, based on their clinical experience, that PNF is superior because it's a form of stretching that more closely approximates "natural" movement.

Your efforts to learn and use this method will be rewarded by greater gains in ROM and flexibility. As more studies are conducted, a clearer picture will emerge to help us understand just what mechanisms are at work in PNF. This clearer understanding will enable us to use PNF stretching even more effectively in the future.

Glossary

abduction: moving a limb away from the midline of the body, as in raising the arm horizontally.

adduction: moving a limb toward the midline of the body, as in lowering the raised arm from a horizontal position.

anterior: toward, located on, or near the front of the body.

concentric contraction: a voluntary contraction in which the muscle shortens as it works.

dorsiflexion: bending the foot upward.

eccentric contraction: a voluntary contraction in which the muscle resists while being lengthened by an outside force; also referred to as "negative work."

eversion: turning the foot so that the sole faces outward.

extension: movement at a joint that increases the joint angle and shifts the parts farther apart, as in straightening the elbow.

flexion: movement at a joint that decreases the joint angle and shifts the parts so that they are closer together, as in bending the elbow.

horizontal abduction: movement of the arm away from the midline of the body, beginning with the arm at shoulder level, as in using the right arm to draw a curtain from left to right.

horizontal adduction: movement of the arm toward the midline of the body, beginning with the arm at shoulder level, as in using the right arm to open a curtain from right to left.

hyperextension: movement of a joint beyond its normal position of extension, as in locking the knees back when standing.

inverse stretch reflex: *see* stretch reflex.

inversion: turning the foot so that the sole faces inward.

isometric contraction: a voluntary muscle contraction in which no movement occurs and the muscle length remains unchanged.

isotonic contraction: a voluntary muscle contraction in which the muscle shortens and which causes joint motion.

lateral: away from the midline.

medial: toward the midline.

myotatic stretch reflex: *see* stretch reflex.

plantarflexion: bending the foot downward.

posterior: toward, located on, or near the rear of the body.

pronation: turning the forearm so the hand faces downward, as in palming a basketball.

prone: lying on the stomach, with the face down.

range of motion: the amount of movement available at a joint, usually expressed in degrees.

reciprocal innervation (reciprocal inhibition): a reflex loop mediated by the muscle spindle cells. When a muscle contracts, reciprocal innervation simultaneously inhibits the opposing muscle. This allows movement to occur around a joint.

rotation: the movement of a bone around its long axis.

stretch reflex: an automatic, involuntary response to stretch that helps protect muscles and joints from injury because of overstretching or excessive strain. In myotatic stretch reflex, when a muscle lengthens too quickly or too far, proprioceptors called muscle spindle cells, located in the belly of the muscle, are stimulated and reflexively cause the muscle to contract. The inverse stretch reflex (also called autogenic inhibition) has the opposite effect of the myotatic stretch reflex. This reflex is mediated by stretch receptors called Golgi tendon organs (GTOs), located in the musculotendinous junction and the tendon. The GTOs monitor the load on the tendon. If the load becomes too great, the GTOs are stimulated. They, in turn, cause the muscle to relax through neurological inhibition.

supinate: to turn the forearm so the hand faces upward, as in holding a bowl of soup.

supine: lying on the back, with the face upward.

References

Anderson, B. 1984. *Stretching*. Bolinas, CA: Shelter.

Beaulieu, J.E. 1981. Developing a stretching program. *Physician and Sports Medicine* 9 (11): 59-69.

Butler, D.S. 1991. *Mobilisation of the nervous system*. New York: Churchill Livingstone.

Chaitow, L. 1996. *Muscle energy techniques*. New York: Churchill Livingstone.

Condon, S.M., and R.S. Hutton. 1987. Soleus muscle electromyographic activity and ankle dorsiflexion range of motion during four stretching procedures. *Physical Therapy* 67: 24-30.

Cornelius, W.L. 1983. Stretch evoked EMG activity by isometric contraction and submaximal concentric contraction. *Athletic Training* 18: 106-9.

Cornelius, W.L., and K. Craft-Hamm. 1988. Proprioceptive neuromuscular facilitation flexibility techniques: Acute effects on arterial blood pressure. *Physician and Sports Medicine* 16(4): 152-61.

Cornelius, W.L., R.L. Jensen, and M.E. Odell. 1995. Effects of PNF stretching phases on acute arterial blood pressure. *Canadian Journal of Applied Physiology* 20(2): 222-29.

Elvey, R.L. 1986. Treatment of arm pain associated with abnormal brachial plexus tension. *Australian Journal of Physiotherapy* 32(4): 225-30.

Etnyre, B.R., and L.D. Abraham. 1986a. Gains in range of ankle dorsiflexion using three popular stretching techniques. *American Journal of Physical Medicine* 65: 189-96.

———. 1986b. H-reflex changes during static stretching and two variations of proprioceptive neuromuscular facilitation techniques. *Electroencephalography and Clinical Neurophysiology* 63 (2): 174-79.

Grant, K.E. 1997. Tender loving care for dancer's legs. *Tactalk*, 22(1) 6-97: 1-5.

Gray, G. 1995. *Lower extremity functional profile*. Adrian, MI: Wynn Marketing, Inc.

Hendrickson, T. 1995. *Manual of orthopedic massage*. Oakland: Author.

Holt, L.E. 1976. *Scientific stretching for sport (3-S)*. Halifax, NS: Sport Research Ltd.

Lucas, R.C., and R. Koslow. 1984. Comparative study of static, dynamic, and proprioceptive neuromuscular facilitation stretching techniques on flexibility. *Perceptual Motor Skills* 58: 615-18.

Mattes, A. 1995. *Active isolated stretching*. Sarasota, FL: Author.

McConnell, J.S. 1986. The management of chondromalacia patella: A long term solution. *Australian Journal of Physiotherapy* 32: 215-23.

Medeiros, J.M., G.L. Smidt, L.F. Burmeister, and G.L. Soderberg. 1977. The influence of isometric exercise and passive stretch on hip joint motion. *Physical Therapy* 57: 518-23.

Moore, M.A., and R.S. Hutton. 1980. Electromyographic investigation of muscle stretching techniques. *Medicine and Science in Sports and Exercise* 12: 322-29.

Myers, T. 1998. Poise: Psoas-piriformis balance. *Massage Magazine* 72 (March/April): 72-83.

Osternig, L., R. Robertson, R. Troxel, and P. Hansen. 1987. Muscle activation during proprioceptive neuromuscular facilitation (PNF) stretching techniques. *American Journal of Physical Medicine* 66: 298-307.

Osternig, L., R. Robertson, R. Troxel, and P. Hansen. 1990. Differential responses to proprioceptive neuromuscular facilitation (PNF) stretch techniques. *Medicine and Science in Sports and Exercise* 22: 106-11.

Prentice, W.E. 1983. A comparison of static stretching and PNF stretching for improving hip joint flexibility. *Athletic Training* 18: 56-59.

Sady, S., M. Wortman, and D. Blanke. 1982. Flexibility training: Ballistic, static or proprioceptive neuromuscular facilitation? *Archives of Physical Medicine and Rehabilitation* 63: 261-63.

Sapega, A.A., T.C. Quedenfeld, R.A. Moyer, and R.A. Butler. 1981. Biophysical factors in range-of-motion exercise. *Physician and Sports Medicine* 9(12): 57-65.

Sherrington, C. 1947. *The integrative action of the nervous system.* 2nd ed. New Haven, CT: Yale University Press.

Surburg, P.R. 1981. Neuromuscular facilitation techniques in sports medicine. *Physician and Sports Medicine* 9 (9): 115-27.

———. 1983. Flexibility exercise re-examined. *Athletic Training* 18: 37-40.

Tanigawa, M.C. 1972. Comparison of the hold-relax procedure and passive mobilization on increasing muscle length. *Physical Therapy* 52: 725-35.

Taylor, D.C., J.D. Dalton, A.V. Seaber, and W.E. Garrett. 1990. Viscoelastic properties of muscle-tendon units: The biomechanical effects of stretching. *American Journal of Sports Medicine* 18: 300-309.

Voss, D., M. Ionta, and B. Myers. 1985. *Proprioceptive neuromuscular facilitation.* 3rd ed. Philadelphia: Harper & Row.

Additional Sources Consulted

Adler, S., D. Beckers, and M. Buck. 1993. *PNF in practice: An illustrated guide.* Berlin: Springer-Verlag.

Alter, M.J. 1996. *Science of flexibility.* 2nd ed. Champaign, IL: Human Kinetics.

Biel, A.R. 1997. *Trail guide to the body.* Boulder, CO: Author.

Blakey, W.P. 1994. *Stretching without pain.* Sechelt, BC: Twin Eagles.

Booher, J.M., and G.A. Thibodeau. 1985. *Athletic injury assessment.* St. Louis: Times Mirror/Mosby.

Cyriax, J.H., and P.J. Cyriax. 1983. *Illustrated manual of orthopaedic medicine.* Boston: Butterworths.

Hoppenfeld, S. 1976. *Physical examination of the spine and extremities.* Norwalk, CT: Appleton-Century-Crofts.

Lockhart, R.D., G.F. Hamilton, and F.W. Fyfe. 1969. *Anatomy of the human body.* 2nd ed. Philadelphia: Lippincott.

Travell, J.G., and D.G. Simons. 1983. *Myofascial pain and dysfunction: The trigger point manual.* Vol. 1. Baltimore: Williams & Wilkins.

———. 1992. *Myofascial pain and dysfunction: The trigger point manual.* Vol. 2. Baltimore: Williams & Wilkins.

Wharton, J., and P. Wharton. 1996. *The stretch book.* New York: Random House.

Index

Note: Italicized page numbers indicate figures.

About the Authors

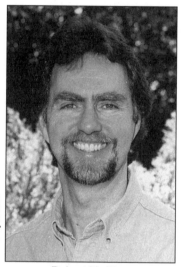

Nancy Hobbs

Robert McAtee

Robert McAtee, BA, LMT, CSCS, has been a sport massage therapist since 1981, specializing in sport and orthopedic massage therapy. He has worked in both clinical settings and private practice and currently maintains a private sport massage practice in Colorado Springs, Colorado.

McAtee teaches facilitated stretching and sport massage seminars throughout the U.S. and internationally to massage therapists, athletic trainers, personal trainers, chiropractors, Olympic-caliber athletes and coaches, and amateur athletes.

McAtee received his massage training at the Institute for Psycho-Structural Balancing in Los Angeles and San Diego (1981) and through the Sports Massage Training Institute (SMTI) in Costa Mesa, California (1986). He is a member of the National Sports Massage Team of the American Massage Therapy Association (AMTA) and is Nationally Certified in Therapeutic Massage and Bodywork. He is a certified strength and conditioning specialist (CSCS) through the National Strength and Conditioning Association (NSCA).

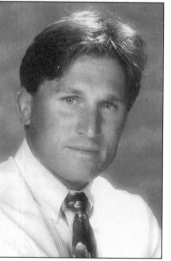

Wendy Pearce Nelson

Jeff Charland

Jeff Charland, PT, ATC, CSCS, GDMT, is a 1983 graduate of the University of Wisconsin at Madison Physical Therapy Program, where he also competed as a varsity athlete on a wrestling scholarship. Since 1987, Charland has lectured in the areas of sports medicine, rehabilitation, and assessment/treatment of neural tissue disorders. He is team trainer and travels internationally with the U.S. Judo and U.S. Wrestling Federations' National and Olympic teams.

Charland completed the graduate program in Manipulative Therapy at Curtin University in Perth, Western Australia, under the direction of Bob Elvey, a world-renowned physiotherapist. He is a certified athletic trainer through the National Athletic Trainers' Association (NATA) and a certified strength and conditioning specialist (CSCS) through the NSCA. In 1997, he earned a certification in Active Release Techniques. He also has served as director of a sports physical therapy clinic in Colorado Springs, Colorado.

For workshops and seminars presented by Bob McAtee, please contact

> Pro-Active Massage Therapy
> 1119 N. Wahsatch Ave, Suite 1
> Colorado Springs, CO 80903
> USA
>
> Tel/Fax: 719-475-1172

or visit his website: **www.stretchman.com**